HIV Treatment Adherence: Challenges for Social Services

HIV Treatment Adherence: Challenges for Social Services has been co-published simultaneously as *Journal of HIV/AIDS & Social Services*, Volume 6, Numbers 1/2 2007.

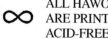

HIV Treatment Adherence: Challenges for Social Services, edited by Lana Sue Ka'opua, PhD, ACSW, LSW, and Nathan L. Linsk, PhD, ACSW (Vol. 6, No. 1/2, 2007). *Examination of the strategies and approaches to help clients to adhere to HIV medication treatments.*

Outreach and Care Approaches to HIV/AIDS Along the US-Mexico Border, edited by Herman Curiel, MSW, PhD, and Helen Land, MSW, PhD (Vol. 5, No. 2, 2006). *Examination of the latest efforts and strategies used to control HIV/AIDS along the US-Mexico Border.*

Midlife and Older Adults and HIV: Implications for Social Service Research, Practice, and Policy, edited by Cynthia Cannon Poindexter, MSW, PhD and Sharon M. Keigher, PhD, MA (Vol. 3, No. 1, 2004). *Introduces policymakers and policy analysts, practitioners in the helping professions, and the public to social services for aging adults living with or affected by HIV/AIDS.*

HIV Treatment Adherence: Challenges for Social Services

Lana Sue Ka'opua, PhD, ACSW, LSW
Nathan L. Linsk, PhD, ACSW
Editors

HIV Treatment Adherence: Challenges for Social Services has been co-published simultaneously as *Journal of HIV/AIDS & Social Services*, Volume 6, Numbers 1/2 2007.

The Haworth Press, Inc.

www.HaworthPress.com

HIV Treatment Adherence: Challenges for Social Services has been
co-published simultaneously as *Journal of HIV/AIDS & Social Services*™,
Volume 6, Numbers 1/2 2007.

Library of Congress Cataloging-in-Publication Data

HIV treatment adherence : challenges for social services / edited by Lana Sue Ka'opua and Nathan L.
Linsk.
        p. ; cm. –has been co-published simultaneously as the (Journal of HIV/AIDS & social ser-
vices ; v 6, no. 1/2)
        Includes bibliographical references and index.
        ISBN-13: 978-0-7890-3626-1 (hard cover : alk. paper)
        1. AIDS (Disease)–Treatment. 2. HIV infections. I. Kao'pua, Lana Sue. II. Linsk, Nathan L.
III. Series.
        [DNLM: 1. HIV Infections–drug therapy. 2. HIV Infections–psychology.
        3. Social Work–methods. 4. Substance-Related Disorders–psychology. 5. Substance-Related
Disorders–therapy. W1 JO671DG v.6 no.1/2 2007 / WC 503.7 H67675 2007]
        RA643.8.H589 2007
        362.196'9792–dc22
                                                                                              2007016365

The HAWORTH PRESS Inc.

Abstracting, Indexing & Outward Linking

PRINT and ELECTRONIC BOOKS & JOURNALS

This section provides you with a list of major indexing & abstracting services and other tools for bibliographic access. That is to say, each service began covering this periodical during the the year noted in the right column. Most Websites which are listed below have indicated that they will either post, disseminate, compile, archive, cite or alert their own Website users with research-based content from this work. (This list is as current as the copyright date of this publication.)

Abstracting, Website/Indexing Coverage . . . . Year When Coverage Began

- ****Academic Search Premier (EBSCO)****
  <http://search.ebscohost.com> 2006

- ****CINAHL (Cumulative Index to Nursing & Allied Health Literature) (EBSCO)**** <http://www.cinahl.com> 2003

- ****CINAHL Plus (EBSCO)****
  <http://search.ebscohost.com>. 2006

- ****Psychological Abstracts (PsycINFO)****
  <http://www.apa.org>. 2006

- ****Social Services Abstracts (Cambridge Scientific Abstracts)****
  <http://www.csa.com> 2006

- ****Social Work Abstracts (NASW)****
  <http://www.silverplatter.com/catalog/swab.htm> 2003

- **(CAB ABSTRACTS, CABI)** <http://www.cabi.org> 2002

- **(IBR) International Bibliography of Book Reviews on the Humanities and Social Sciences (Thomson)**
  <http://www.saur.de>. 2006

- **(IBZ) International Bibliography of Periodical Literature on the Humanities and Social Sciences (Thomson)**
  <http://www.saur.de>. 2002

(continued)

(continued)

(continued)

Bibliographic Access

Special Bibliographic Notes related to special journal issues
(separates) and indexing/abstracting:

- indexing/abstracting services in this list will also cover material in any "separate" that is co-published simultaneously with Haworth's special thematic journal issue or DocuSerial. Indexing/abstracting usually covers material at the article/chapter level.
- monographic co-editions are intended for either non-subscribers or libraries which intend to purchase a second copy for their circulating collections.
- monographic co-editions are reported to all jobbers/wholesalers/approval plans. The source journal is listed as the "series" to assist the prevention of duplicate purchasing in the same manner utilized for books-in-series.
- to facilitate user/access services all indexing/abstracting services are encouraged to utilize the co-indexing entry note indicated at the bottom of the first page of each article/chapter/contribution.
- this is intended to assist a library user of any reference tool (whether print, electronic, online, or CD-ROM) to locate the monographic version if the library has purchased this version but not a subscription to the source journal.
- individual articles/chapters in any Haworth publication are also available through the Haworth Document Delivery Service (HDDS).

As part of Haworth's continuing committment to better serve our library patrons, we are proud to be working with the following electronic services:

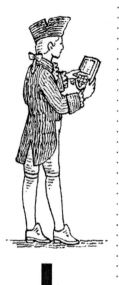

AGGREGATOR SERVICES

EBSCOhost

Ingenta

J-Gate

Minerva

OCLC FirstSearch

Oxmill

SwetsWise

EBSCO HOST

INF-RMATICS

Ingenta

J-Gate

MINERVA

FirstSearch

information to empower
Oxmill Publishing

SwetsWise

LINK RESOLVER SERVICES

1Cate (Openly Informatics)

CrossRef

Gold Rush (Coalliance)

LinkOut (PubMed)

LINKplus (Atypon)

LinkSolver (Ovid)

LinkSource with A-to-Z (EBSCO)

Resource Linker (Ulrich)

SerialsSolutions (ProQuest)

SFX (Ex Libris)

Sirsi Resolver (SirsiDynix)

Tour (TDnet)

Vlink (Extensity, formerly Geac)

WebBridge (Innovative Interfaces)

1cate

crossref

Gold Rush

LinkOut.
LINKING TO A WORLD OF RESOURCES

atypon

A to Z
EBSCO

O V I D   LinkSolver

ULRICH'S
RESOURCE LINKER

S·F·X

SerialsSolutions

SirsiDynix

TOUR

extensity

WebBridge

HIV Treatment Adherence: Challenges for Social Services

CONTENTS

ABOUT THE EDITORS

Lana Sue Ka'opua, PhD, ACSW, LSW, is Associate Professor at the University of Hawai`i School of Social Work and at the Cancer Research Center of Hawai`i. As a practitioner, she has extensive experience in health/behavioral health clinics located in medically underserved communities. As an educator, she teaches courses in health and social work, research methods, and social work practice. For over a decade, Dr. Ka'opua has conducted research and training in HIV with special foci on treatment adherence and culturally responsive social service interventions. Her current research emphasizes interventions to eliminate cancer and other health disparities. She is principal investigator of an NIH-funded project to increase adherence to routine mammography guidelines among medically underserved Native Hawaiian women and serves as co-investigator on a CDC-funded project to develop a model for improving technical assistance, funding support, and data collection in the U.S.-Associated Pacific Island nations of Micronesia.

Nathan L. Linsk, PhD, ACSW, is Professor at the Jane Addams College of Social Work at the University of Illinois at Chicago. Dr. Linsk established and is Principal Investigator for the seven state Midwest AIDS Training and Education Center and co-Principal Investigator on the six state Great Lakes Addictions Technology Transfer Center, which provide training, technical assistance and capacity building to both providers and care systems in the addictions and HIV fields. Dr. Linsk conducts research and develops service programs related to family caregiving issues, program evaluation, case management systems development and health professional training. He has authored over 45 articles and four books. He heads the evaluation team for the Chicago Department of Health Ryan White CARE Title I Services, which has established service standards quality improvement models to do quality assurance and also evaluates service needs and outcomes. Dr. Linsk has shared leadership for the Social Work Education in Ethiopia Partnership helping establish the first MSW and PhD social work education programs in Ethiopia. He was an African AIDS Regional Research Fulbright Fellow in Ethiopia in 2006, studying the role of non-governmental organizations in decision-making and community support for antiretroviral HIV medications. He is Principal Investigator on an HIV Twinning Center project partnering the Jane Addams College of Social Work and the Institute of Social Work Dar es Salaam, Tanzania to develop competencies to serve orphans and vulnerable children related to HIV. Dr. Linsk has served as co-Editor of the *Journal of HIV/AIDS & Social Services* since its inception.

Introduction:
Addressing Challenges of Adherence to HIV Medications for Social Services Practice, Research, and Training

Highly Active Antiretroviral Therapy (HAART) can significantly improve the health outcomes of people living with HIV. Documented to suppress the rate of viral replication in the body to undetectable levels, decrease incidence of opportunistic infections, and delay AIDS progression, HAART offers the prospect of living longer with an enhanced quality of life. Although treatments are efficacious, individual benefits rely on near-perfect adherence or steady devotion to follow medication regimen as prescribed. These complex regimens have been difficult for many to manage.

PSYCHOSOCIAL/SPIRITUAL CHALLENGES

Achieving high levels of adherence often requires navigating a sea of daunting psychosocial/spiritual challenges, as well as bio-medical ones. For persons prescribed combination antiretroviral regimen, the psychosocial/spiritual challenges are considerable and include: (1) integrating complex regimen into daily life, (2) staying motivated to consistently take regimen for indefinite periods of time, (3) living with treatment side-effects that may compromise capacity to enjoy deeply

[Haworth co-indexing entry note]: "Introduction: Addressing Challenges of Adherence to HIV Medications for Social Services Practice, Research, and Training." Ka'opua, Lana Sue, and 'Nathan L. Linsk. Co-published simultaneously in *the Journal of HIV/AIDS & Social Services* (The Haworth Press, Inc.) Vol. 6, No. 1/2, 2007, pp. 1-8; and: *HIV Treatment Adherence: Challenges for Social Services* (ed: Lana Sue Ka'opua and Nathan L. Linsk) The Haworth Press, Inc., 2007, pp. 1-8. Single or multiple copies of this article are available for a fee from The Haworth Document Delivery Service [1-800-HAWORTH, 9:00 a.m. - 5:00 p.m. (EST). E-mail address: docdelivery@haworthpress.com].

Available online at http://jhaso.haworthpress.com
doi: 10.1300/J187v06n01_01

valued, culturally-patterned activities, (4) finding the inner fortitude to deal with the perceived stigma related to HIV or taking HIV medications as well as uncertainty and lifestyle accommodations which ensue when regimens are modified, and (5) using personal strengths, social support and spiritual resources to meet these challenges and sustain quality of life. These challenges are further complicated by co-occurring substance abuse, depression, and other health/behavioral health conditions, as well as the need for health resources such as housing, social support, adequate nutrition, and adherence-specific assistance.

The challenges of adherence to HAART have not changed since the inception of combination antiretroviral regimens nearly a decade ago. Recent developments have brought both good news and ongoing challenges. Since HAART began treatment options have greatly expanded, dosage frequency and pill burden are reduced, and required adherence levels may vary by treatment regimen (King, Brun, & Kempf, 2005; Maggiolo et al., 2005) making adherence more feasible for many. The prospects of medications for the rest of one's life may contribute to adherence fatigue and the need for ongoing supports. However, there are also many promising developments in knowledge and technologies *by and for* those in social services which may effectively support clients to mediate the challenges of initiating and sustaining steady devotion to HAART regimens.

DEVELOPMENTS IN SOCIAL SERVICES PRACTICE, RESEARCH, AND TRAINING

This special volume focuses on knowledge, strategies, and approaches relevant to supporting treatment adherence. Contributors are psychosocial researchers, social workers and other social service practitioners, educators, and policy advocates in the advanced theatre of HIV and HAART intervention. These contributors represent diverse disciplinary perspectives, yet share a committed vision to deepening understanding and more effectively addressing issues related to optimal adherence, as experienced by diverse consumer groups.

Featured in this issue are a rich and comprehensive collection of articles. We begin with an assessment of the state of the field and a global overview. In an invited article, Stirratt and Gordon highlight major themes emerging from *The 1st Annual International Conference on HIV Treatment Adherence*. Identified and briefly discussed are adherence interventions found efficacious in randomized clinical trials and clinical and research approaches for effective assessment of adherence. Against this hopeful backdrop are identified future directions for translating research from the bench of discovery to clinical and community settings, for addressing needs to expand treatment access, and for coordinated and integrated service delivery. While progress has been made in approaches and technologies for initiating adherence regimens, attention is now needed to developing evidence-based methods for sustaining adherence. The role of social service practitioners, researchers, and educators is critical in meeting these evolving challenges.

The following articles address a very important set of themes about the current status of adherence research and practice.

Psychosocial/Spiritual Predictors of HAART Adherence

Knowledge of factors predicting adherence is essential to an assessment of treatment readiness and to delivery of supportive interventions across the HIV trajectory. To this end, four papers focus on identifying predictors:

- Gruber, Sorensen, and Haug review adherence predictors from 17 prospective studies qualified by their methodological rigor. Across all studies, the most robust predictor of optimal adherence was stable housing and consistently associated with low adherence was use of stimulants. The need for multi-disciplinary and inter-organizational collaboration is indicated to address structural barriers and provide supportive resources at the intersection of HIV and co-occurring substance use.
- Hamilton, Razzano, and Martin focus their inquiry on specific sources of social support among ethnically diverse clients. Their sample was drawn from clients simultaneously enrolled in a medication adherence study and a local AIDS service organization. Source of support was found to be most relevant to adherence. Specifically, functional support from partners consistently predicted adherence across time and regardless of ethnicity. Family support was reported frequently by clients of color and tended to be perceived as positive. Interestingly, family support predicted lower levels of adherence and was associated with more missed doses and reasons for non-adherence. The authors provide a compelling discussion of this and other results. Indicated is the need for interventions that address clients' diverse support networks.

- Pomeroy, Thompson, Gober, and Noel conducted a pilot study of adherence predictors relevant to Fisher's Information-Motivation-Behavior Model of HIV Prevention. Multivariate analysis of survey data from an ethnically representative sample of HIV positive adults indicate that Fisher's model may be relevant for predicting adherence and suggests the potentially important link between prevention and treatment support. These authors note the need for a more extensive examination of ethnicity and adherence to more precisely inform development of culturally competent interventions for ethnically diverse client groups.

- Sunil and McGehee report findings on the relationship of adherence and social and religious support among HIV positive clients of diverse ethnic groups. Based on a secondary analysis of survey data from a nationally representative sample, the relationship of adherence to support varied by ethnic group membership. While religious and social support predicted better adherence among African Americans and Hispanic clients, sociodemographic characteristics such as education and age predicted adherence among Whites. Results indicate the need for differential and possibly culturally appropriate strategies to improve adherence outcomes among diverse client groups. Partnerships with religious organizations are suggested as a potentially promising strategy for encouraging adherence among African American and Hispanic clients.

Social Service Interventions

Two articles present results from research to develop adherence counseling interventions that are informed by empirical and practice wisdom. Results from these developmental studies are promising for social service providers seeking to enhance client adherence through similar programs. Practice-relevant guidelines are offered.

- Cooperman, Parsons, Chabon, Berg, and Arnsten developed an adherence counseling program tailored to clients with HIV and co-occurring opiod dependence. Motivational interviewing and cognitive-behavioral skills training were used by paraprofessional counselors in a limited-term intervention. Results from this feasibility study indicate that paraprofessional counselors trained in these modalities may be important, even critical partners to social workers and other health/behavioral health professionals involved in supporting client adherence.

- Scheid, in conjunction with social work and nursing professionals, developed a specialized adherence counseling and education program which was evaluated for feasibility in a self-selected sample of HIV positive clients. Adherence was assessed through multiple measures at two points of follow-up. Results indicate that adherence generally improved. Social support, assistance in navigating adherence barriers, and demonstration of unconditional positive regard were viewed by staff as important program components. Such a program integrated into existing social work and/or case management services may be feasible.

Provider Training

Increasingly recognized is the need for integrative models of social service practice which address the varied and multiple challenges associated with ART adherence in cost-effective ways. Increasing the capacity of service providers to do this may be optimally accomplished through systematic training anchored in methods of adult pedagogy.

- Bass, Linsk, and Mitchell evaluated a training program intended to enhance substance abuse counselors' (SAC) capacity and comfort in providing adherence-related counseling. Pedagogical methods involved the use of case scenarios and client simulation. Changes occurring as a result of training were assessed prior to training, immediately following training, and at five-month post-training follow-up. SAC were receptive to medication-related education and as a result of completing training, reported being more comfortable in discussing sensitive adherence-related issues. Client advocacy with a physician remained an area of less comfort.

Voices from People Living with HIV and HAART

The lived experience of adherence to HAART is influenced by many factors which may not be adequately captured by conventional empirical research using quantitative methods of data collection and analysis.

Crucial to consider is the holistic experience of those living with HIV and medication adherence.

- Gilbert, Abel, Stewart, and Zilberman report on facilitating and disabling factors to adherence as based on statements elicited from 90 individuals living with HIV and co-occurring substance use. Consumer statements provide a rich description of the range and complexity of adherence factors beyond substance use and emphasize the need for social support, knowledge, and assistance in coping with fear and mistrust. This report may serve to sensitize practitioners and researchers to perspectives and service needs which might not otherwise be considered.

OUR WORK IN ADDRESSING
ADHERENCE CHALLENGES

HIV/AIDS care and services reinforce many lessons we have learned in providing comprehensive continuing care to a range of client populations. Helping clients focus on adherence, whether it be to medication regimens or other parts of the treatment plan, taps the unique skills of psychosocial assessment, behavioral and social interventions, and interventions that address systems and policy issues which derive from the basis of providing humane social services. While social workers, case managers, nurses, psychologists and others may take on unique adherence counseling roles, HIV work has been and continues to be characterized by the need for collaboration and team work (Willinger & Rice, 2003). Our work is highly characterized by multi-disciplinary and inter-organizational collaboration to address structural barriers and provide supportive resources at the intersections of HIV and co-occurring conditions including substance use, mental health and the evolving array of other medical conditions that occur as people live longer with HIV (e.g., hypertension, diabetes and cardiovascular problems).

Moreover, HIV care and services can only be effective within the entire spectrum of HIV intervention including education, prevention and treatment support. As efforts to focus both on primary prevention and prevention for people who are HIV positive (Centers for Disease Control and Prevention [CDC], 1997) have revealed, prevention of transmission goes hand-in-hand with prevention of further complications and co-existing conditions. Helping clients to adhere to medications and care plans utilizes the same underlying behavioral change methodologies as do prevention and health promotion strategies. Furthermore, it is essential that the roles of service providers be directed not only toward individual clients but also toward families and communities. The latter is especially true in supporting adherence among ethno-culturally diverse client groups and their support networks.

To address needs of people living with HIV, including treatment adherence, we have come to understand the benefits of case managers to assist with ensuring that the plan of care is sufficient, that effective linkages between organizations and programs be sustained, that required social supports are present, and that the client has access to advocacy support. Clients may benefit from an array of expertise ranging from the highly skilled clinician through the case manager, paraprofessional counselors and volunteer "buddies," particularly when there is an acute crisis or late stage care.

As these articles point out, adherence programs are often integrated into existing clinic programs, social work and/or case management services. These integrative models of social service practice may address the varied and multiple challenges associated with medication adherence.

After more than twenty-five years of this epidemic and in the absence of a vaccine or cure, much can be done to sustain length and quality of life. While research has emerged that is useful, this research must be translated into educational and service programs to ensure that providers utilize emerging best practices. Treatment access continues to be critical and with compressing resources allocated at Federal and State levels, continued advocacy is necessary. Because these medications are meant to be taken over the life course, advocacy to ensure access, necessarily must be viewed as ongoing and protracted over the long-term. Of course, the need for continued access is even more critical on the international arena.

As noted by C. Everett Koop, former U.S. Surgeon General, medications work only when they are taken. For adherence to HAART, this means that medications must be taken on schedule, under correct conditions, and importantly, supported by the partnership between the client and the health providers, the latter of who optimally work together in collaborated and coordinated ways. Assessing treatment readiness, implementing HAART, ensuring activation of the psychosocial/spiritual supports needed to sustain adherence, and addressing the ongoing needs of those in care continue to be our challenges. However, these challenges may be effectively addressed by the diverse intervention models and increasingly, integrated service programs which have evolved.

Lana Sue Ka'opua, PhD, ACSW, LSW
School of Social Work
University of Hawai`i-Manoa

Nathan L. Linsk, PhD, ACSW
Jane Addams College of Social Work
University of Illinois at Chicago

REFERENCES

Centers for Disease Control and Prevention (1997). HIV prevention case management–literature review and current practice. Retrieved October 7, 2006 at http://www.cdc.gov/hiv/topics/prev_prog/CRCS/resources/PCML/index.htm.

King, M. S., Brun, S. C., & Kempf, D. J. (2005). Relationship between adherence and the development of resistance in antiretroviral-naive, HIV-1-infected patients receiving lopinavir/ritonavir or nelfinavir. *Journal of Infectious Diseases, 191*, 2046-2052.

Maggiolo, F., Ravasio, L., Ripamonti, D., Gregis, G., Quinzan, G., Arici, C. et al. (2005). Similar adherence rates favor different virologic outcomes for patients treated with nonnucleoside analogues or protease inhibitors. *Clinical Infectious Diseases, 40*, 158-163.

Willinger, B. I., & Rice, A. (Eds.) (2003). A History of AIDS Social Work in Hospitals: A Daring Response to an Epidemic. New York, NY: The Haworth Press.

doi:10.1300/J187v06n01_01

INVITED ARTICLE

HIV Treatment Adherence Research and Intervention: Current Advances and Future Challenges

Michael J. Stirratt, PhD
Christopher M. Gordon, PhD

SUMMARY. Maximizing treatment adherence is essential for optimizing clinical outcomes among HIV/AIDS patients. A decade after the introduction of combination antiretroviral therapy (ART), numerous achievements and continued challenges are evident within research on HIV treatment adherence. In this paper, we illustrate some key themes within current treatment adherence research by highlighting presentations from a recent conference focused on this topic (the 2006 NIMH/IAPAC International Conference on HIV Treatment Adherence). We then discuss

Michael J. Stirratt, PhD, is Program Officer for the Adherence Program and Christopher M. Gordon, PhD, is the Chief of the Secondary Prevention and Translational Research Branch at the Center for Mental Health Research on AIDS, Division of AIDS and Health and Behavior Research, National Institute of Mental Health.

Address correspondence to: Dr. Stirratt, DAHBR, National Institute of Mental Health, MSC 9619, 6001 Executive Boulevard, Bethesda, MD 20892 (E-mail: stirrattm @mail.nih.gov).

[Haworth co-indexing entry note]: "HIV Treatment Adherence Research and Intervention: Current Advances and Future Challenges." Stirratt, Michael J., and Christopher M. Gordon. Co-published simultaneously in *the Journal of HIV/AIDS & Social Services* (The Haworth Press, Inc.) Vol. 6, No. 1/2, 2007, pp. 9-22; and: *HIV Treatment Adherence: Challenges for Social Services* (ed: Lana Sue Ka'opua and Nathan L. Linsk) The Haworth Press, Inc., 2007, pp. 9-22. Single or multiple copies of this article are available for a fee from The Haworth Document Delivery Service [1-800-HAWORTH, 9:00 a.m. - 5:00 p.m. (EST). E-mail address: docdelivery@haworthpress.com].

several ongoing challenges confronting the field, and suggest that multi-disciplinary research will be essential for overcoming these challenges and strengthening our efforts to improve and sustain adherence to HIV treatment. doi:10.1300/J187v06n01_02 *[Article copies available for a fee from The Haworth Document Delivery Service: 1-800-HAWORTH. E-mail address: <docdelivery@haworthpress.com> Website: <http://www.HaworthPress.com> © 2007 by The Haworth Press, Inc. All rights reserved.]*

KEYWORDS. HIV/AIDS, adherence, antiretroviral therapy, HAART, ART, intervention

INTRODUCTION

Effective treatment for HIV/AIDS is broadly available within developed nations in the form of combination antiretroviral therapy (ART). However, the full benefits of these drugs are not realized in many HIV seropositive (HIV+) patients due to the challenges of maintaining high levels of treatment adherence. Research documents that medication adherence is the strongest predictor of viral suppression (Arnsten et al., 2001; Bangsberg et al., 2000; Paterson et al., 2000), progression to AIDS (Bangsberg et al., 2001), and mortality (Garcia de Olalla et al., 2002; Hogg et al., 2002). Although new studies have recently indicated that more potent drug regimens may allow for effective viral suppression at lower levels of adherence (Maggiolo et al., 2005; Bangsberg, 2006; King, Brun, & Kempf, 2005), it is important to emphasize that improving adherence to any degree can only increase the likelihood of suppressing the virus and postponing disease progression. Striving for the highest possible level of adherence therefore remains essential to optimizing HIV treatment outcomes (Gulick, 2006).

Towards this end, the National Institutes of Health (NIH) supports a substantial portfolio of research aimed at understanding and enhancing HIV treatment adherence. The National Institute of Mental Health (NIMH) supports a number of interdisciplinary projects that draw upon the expertise and skills of all treatment team members–providers, nurses, case managers, mental health professionals, pharmacists, other staff members who provide ancillary services, patients, and researchers. This special collection underscores the important role that social service providers have in supporting HIV treatment adherence, so we are pleased to contribute to an excellent set of papers that will reach this audience. In this invited article, we offer a brief review of current trends in HIV adherence research, highlighting a new conference opportunity that social service providers may consider for sharing their experiences and advancing their understandings and approaches to adherence. We then conclude with a discussion of the ongoing challenges facing the field.

TAKING STOCK:
REPORT FROM THE 1ST INTERNATIONAL CONFERENCE
ON HIV TREATMENT ADHERENCE

In collaboration with a broad set of governmental agencies and professional organizations, the 1st Annual International Conference on HIV Treatment Adherence was held in March 2006. The conference was designed to provide a unique forum for the presentation and discussion of state-of-the science in HIV treatment adherence research, as well as current behavioral and clinical perspectives in practicum. Approximately 350 physicians, nurses, social workers, mental health professionals, pharmacists, behavioral researchers, social scientists and other providers attended the conference in Jersey City, New Jersey (across from Manhattan). The agenda for the conference successfully brought together programs and perspectives from 20 countries. Slide presentations from plenary addresses and oral presentations (referred to below) can be found at <http://www.iapac.org/home.asp?pid=6514>, a website hosted by a co-convener of the conference, the International Association of Physicians in AIDS Care (IAPAC). Abstracts for the oral and poster presentations have also been published (NIMH/IAPAC, 2006a, 2006b, 2006c). The 2nd Conference is scheduled for March 28-30, 2007, at the same location.

Although the conference presentations detailed numerous approaches for improving and sustaining patient adherence, we highlight only a small set of central themes addressed within the conference. The first theme could be described as "intervention works." Conference presenter Jane Simoni shared the results of the first meta-analysis of randomized controlled trials (RCTs) of interventions for adherence to antiretroviral therapy for HIV (Simoni, Pearson, Pantalone, Crepaz, & Marks, 2006). Across 19 RCT studies with more than 1,800 participants, those who received an adherence intervention were 1.5 times as likely to report 95% adherence and 1.25 times as likely to achieve an undetectable viral load than participants in comparison conditions. This was a welcome message for conference participants who are eager to implement efficacious interventions with their patients. It is notable that a range of modalities and intensities of interventions demonstrated efficacy–so a menu of options is available for providers in order to choose a program that suits their setting. A next major step for the field will be to work together to develop systems to facilitate adoption of such interventions in practice. This translational challenge is discussed in more detail later in this article.

In addition to this summary presentation, numerous conference presentations from individual studies and settings underscored the theme of effective intervention by describing proven or promising approaches for promoting adherence. For example, an innovative case management approach was offered by Christopher Mitchell, who presented preliminary findings from an ongoing adherence intervention study conducted with marginally-housed HIV+ clients (Mitchell, Freels, Creticos, & Douglas, 2006). The program, entitled DAART+, integrates a modified version of Directly Observed Therapy (DOT) with HIV risk reduction counseling. The intervention is administered through multiple phases: an initial assessment of client readiness to initiate ART, three months of intensive (daily) meetings to observe client ART adherence, and then tapered (twice weekly) meetings to monitor adherence. The goal is to help clients adopt and autonomously maintain long-term medication adherence and HIV risk reduction behaviors. Initial findings from a pilot intervention conducted with 30 clients were promising, in that large proportions of participants demonstrated improved CD4 counts and decreased viral loads over a nine-month follow-up assessment period. This work offers important innovations by systematically addressing client readiness for ART, tapering DOT to promote eventual independent medication adherence, and behavioral risk reduction. Other examples of intervention-focused presentation included Robert Remien, who provided a tutorial on an effective couples-based intervention to support patient ART adherence (Remien, Stirratt, & Dognin, 2006), and Victoria Mitrani, who discussed the use of Structural Ecosystems Therapy to promote medication adherence in HIV+ African American women (Feaster, Mitrani, Prado, & Szapocznik, 2006).

A second conference theme related to clinical and research assessment of adherence. A wide variety of approaches for assessing adherence are available, including pill count, self-report, electronic monitoring (MEMS caps), and therapeutic drug monitoring. Presenter Ann Kurth reviewed these methods and discussed their comparative utility and validity in adherence research (Kurth, 2006). Sharon Mannheimer described an innovative three-item assessment of patient ART adherence entitled the CASE index (Mannheimer et al., 2006). The index was designed for quick and simple administration with patients in clinic or service settings, and study results showed strong concurrence between responses to the index and standard patient three-day self-reports of adherence, as well as correspondence with patient viral load. In this and other presentations, advances in the utility and validity of clinician and researcher assessment of patient adherence were observed.

A third conference theme focused on international HIV treatment adherence research and initiatives. The unprecedented global initiative for HIV treatment access within developing nations has received much emphasis and is beginning to bring ART to those in greatest need. Although much has been written about how HIV prevention should accompany treatment rollout (e.g., Valdiserri, 2004), it has not been as clear that expansion and integration of adherence interventions in these countries is viewed as essential. At this conference, the message was clear. Presenters and attendees were unanimous regarding the importance of supporting and sustaining high adherence in the context of expanded treatment access. Presenter Peter Mugyenyi identified ART adherence as one of the most important challenges facing the ongoing treatment rollout in Africa (Mugyenyi, 2006). Noting concerns that adherence may decline as treatment is more widely available, he presented a model for a coordinated approach for supporting adherence across many clinics in Uganda that can be tailored to patient needs and flexibly adjusted in the face of numerous structural barriers. Their system for monitoring and intervention could serve as an example for both developed and developing nations. Other conference presenters, including David Bangsberg and Norma Ware (Bangsberg, Simoni, Ware, & Castro, 2006), discussed the importance of developing theoretical models of adherence that can guide culturally appropriate and effective intervention in resource-limited settings.

LOOKING AHEAD:
FUTURE CHALLENGES IN HIV TREATMENT ADHERENCE

To strengthen and sustain approaches for maintaining high treatment adherence among HIV+ patients, future research initiatives, service provision, and policymaking will need to address and overcome a number of critical challenges. We offer the following considerations for discussion, and do so with the recognition that there are many additional and important directions for the field to pursue that cannot be fully detailed here.

Future approaches to promoting HIV treatment adherence face the challenge of not only improving patient adherence, but also sustaining patient adherence over a lifetime. As indicated by the Simoni et al. (2006) meta-analysis described above, existing intervention studies have clearly demonstrated efficacy in improving patient adherence and clinical outcomes. However, the meta-analytic results were limited to data collected either immediately post-intervention or at the first follow-up assessment, and the average length of time for follow-up was only 60 days. In many randomized clinical trials of adherence interventions that employ longer periods of follow-up assessment, initial intervention effects typically decline with time, often to the point where rates of ART adherence are indistinguishable between treatment and control groups after a six month period. The next generation of adherence research, services, and policy will need to identify and promote innovative methods for maintenance of patient adherence. This may involve the use of booster sessions, new technologies, and the direct integration of adherence support into ongoing care, among other approaches. Documenting longer-term impacts on adherence behavior may also require alternative research designs and methodologies that incorporate extended follow-up periods.

To help sustain adherence, future research and intervention could consider greater emphasis on the role of social and structural factors. Although the growing adherence research literature has identified a variety of factors that can impede and facilitate adherence to HIV treatment, most of this work has addressed individual-level factors such as patient knowledge, motivation, cognitive deficits, and mood states. These are essential considerations, but emerging findings from studies conducted in domestic and international settings are now bringing greater attention to broader, multi-level influences on adherence behavior. These influences represent multiple aspects of social networks and structural environments, including societal HIV/AIDS stigma and interpersonal HIV serostatus disclosure (e.g., Golin, Isasi, Bontempi, & Eng, 2002; Kidder et al., 2006; Peretti-Watel et al., 2006; Rintamaki, Davis, Skripkaukas, Bennett, & Wolf, 2006; Stirratt et al., 2006), as well as institutional and economic factors, such as access to adequate and affordable transportation, food, housing, and health care (e.g., Crane et al., 2006; Weiser et al., 2003). These emerging considerations will require fresh approaches to the design and implementation of effective HIV treatment adherence interventions.

From our perspective, researchers will also need to broaden the scope of interventions to enhance HIV treatment adherence. To date, studies have principally targeted patient adherence to the dosage requirements for ART. This work will always hold critical importance, since ART regimens generally demand strong adherence to optimize their clinical benefits. However, other facets of ART adherence have received less attention and may make important contributions to patient care and clinical outcomes. For example, persistent racial and ethnic disparities in ART initiation among eligible patients must be addressed (Gebo et al., 2004; Palacio, Kahn, Richards, & Morin, 2002; Stone, 2004). Another consideration is that notable proportions of patients who initiate ART discontinue their treatment within two years due to side effects, virologic failure, or psychosocial concerns (Ahdieh-Grant et al., 2001, 2005; Mocroft et al., 2001). These ART discontinuations have been associated with deleterious clinical outcomes, particularly in patients with limited immune reconstitution (Touloumi et al., 2006). Interventions designed to prevent unsupervised or inopportune treatment discontinuations in vulnerable patients would be helpful. Such programs could separately or simultaneously target patient preparation to initiate therapy, the selection of tolerable regimens, effective management of side effects, continuous access to prescription refills, and the maintenance of strong adherence over time, among other factors. In one tested approach, Frick and colleagues found that multidisciplinary adherence counseling from an integrated clinic treatment team significantly extended the amount of time that patients remained on ART without interruption (Frick, Tapia, Grant, Novotny, & Kerzee, 2006).

Adopting a broad, multidimensional understanding of HIV treatment adherence also argues for addressing important aspects of patient care other than ART. Many patients never initiate care after testing HIV seropositive, and those who enroll in HIV treatment often do not attend enough medical appointments to benefit (Giordano et al., 2005). In addition, many HIV+ patients have unmet needs for services such as housing, public assistance, and psychiatric treatment, and these unmet needs have been associated with decreased likelihood of ART use and poor ART adherence (Reif, Whetten, Lowe, & Ostermann, 2006). To complement the ongoing research on adherence to ART medications, innovative interventions to increase consistent utilization of HIV care and social services are needed. In a recent randomized clinical trial, a case management intervention to enhance linkage to HIV care among newly-diagnosed persons with HIV demonstrated efficacy (Gardner et al., 2005). Compared to standard of care, a higher proportion of patients in the case management condition (60% vs. 78%) reported seeing an HIV provider at least once within 6 months. Future research could therefore aid patient care and clinical outcomes by addressing linkage to treatment, consistent attendance at medical appointments, and follow-through on referrals, such as to mental health services, substance abuse treatment, and other social services.

Studies are also needed that will further document and capitalize upon the intersections between HIV treatment adherence and HIV prevention. Recent years have brought increasing recognition of "prevention for positives" as a key component of comprehensive HIV prevention in the U.S. (Janssen et al., 2001). This necessarily involves behavioral interventions and risk reduction counseling, but treatment adherence also has a role to play. Adherence to ART treatment can yield reductions in viral load that are associated with reduced infectivity and HIV transmission, even after controlling for safer sex practices (Castilla et al., 2005; Kayitenkore et al., 2006). Interventions to promote widespread treatment uptake and strong ART adherence among HIV seropositive individuals could therefore produce decreases in HIV transmission and new infections on a population level (Montaner et al., 2006; Velasco-Hernandez, Gershengorn, & Blower, 2002). At the same time, some studies suggest that patients who are least adherent to ART regimens are also the least adherent to safer sex practices (Kalichman & Rompa, 2003). This confluence suggests that simultaneous attention to both issues may help to prevent transmission of drug resistant viral strains to uninfected individuals. Future initiatives are indicated to integrate risk reduction counseling and adherence interventions into the provision of primary care and services for HIV+ individuals. In addition, emerging medication-based prevention tools targeted to HIV seronegative individuals, such as post-exposure prophylaxis ([PEP]; Centers for Disease Control and Prevention [CDC], 2005; Omrani & Freedman, 2005) and pre-exposure prophylaxis ([PrEP]; Liu, Grant, & Buchbinder, 2006; Youle & Wainberg, 2003) present new domains where understanding and promoting medication adherence may be critical for preventing new HIV infections.

Among the most pressing challenges facing research on HIV treatment adherence involve the efforts to translate research results into clinical practice. A decade of research on HIV treatment adherence has produced a modest clinical and behavioral armamentarium that includes greatly simplified medication regimens and a growing set of behavioral interventions that demonstrate short-term efficacy. Providers in the U.S. and abroad are in immediate need of these evidence-based interventions for their patients and clients, and clinicians and social workers need guidance regarding which interventions are appropriate for which patients. Little is known about contextual issues that affect intervention adoption, adaptation, and effectiveness of adherence interventions that were tested in randomized clinical trials (RCTs). Organizational leadership, clinic personnel turnover, and organizational size are factors that may influence implementation of new interventions (Gandelman & Rietmeijer, 2004). An additional consideration for research is that, whether intentional or unintentional, interventions will be modified in real-world settings. The effectiveness of HIV treatment adherence interventions implemented outside of rigorous RCTs may rely on how well fidelity to the intervention protocols can be maintained in the face of competing clinic demands. How best to measure success in translational research also needs examination; success could be defined as whether or not an intervention is adopted and sustained for a specified time period, and/or success could be measured through direct assessment of patient outcomes.

Finally, it is critical to fully "internationalize" HIV treatment adherence research and intervention. After a decade of HAART, to our knowledge the only published adherence RCTs have been conducted in North America and Europe. Outside of these regions, in both developed and developing countries where HIV treatment is becoming more widely available, even descriptive data and studies of adherence predictors are in their early stages. Without rapid attention to adherence internationally, decisions about adherence interventions to accompany treatment will be made in the absence of empirical support. We do not mean to suggest that important work has not been conducted, just that more is urgently needed. It is remarkable that even in the absence of significant support, influential models for HIV treatment and adherence have been developed within resource-constrained settings, and collaboration with communities has been essential. For example, in Haiti, accompagnateurs play an important role in patients' adherence to treatment (Farmer et al., 2001; Koenig, Leandre, & Farmer, 2004). Variations of this model, using peers or community health workers, are now being tested in other international (Sarna et al., 2006) and U.S. settings (Behforouz, Farmer, & Mukherjee, 2004). Because so little is known about adherence in many international settings, recommendations for research directions will not be as specific as the suggestions cited earlier. Rather, it is sufficient to conclude that nearly *all* aspects would benefit from further research as soon as possible.

A decade of research on HIV treatment adherence has produced many advances. Within some settings, there has been an articulation of the fundamental barriers, facilitators, and factors associated with ART adherence (e.g., Ammassari et al., 2002; Fogarty et al., 2002). Further, a rapidly increasing set of interventions that are effective in improving adherence has been developed (Simoni et al., 2006). However, as identified in this article, many challenges continue to confront our efforts to optimize patient adherence to HIV treatment. It is difficult to envision how these challenges can be effectively addressed without strong inter-disciplinary and multi-stakeholder collaboration. HIV treatment adherence is a multifaceted phenomenon that necessarily implicates aspects of biology, pharmacology, medicine, behavioral science, epidemiology, and sociology. Comprehensive understandings and effective approaches for maximizing patient adherence will therefore require contributions and collaborations across multiple disciplines. This importantly includes the social workers, case managers, treatment advocates, health care administrators, and mental health professionals who provide a broad range of essential services and support for HIV+ clients. We are pleased with the contribution that this special volume makes to this ongoing dialogue, and we invite continued participation and collaboration on interdisciplinary research that will help sustain HIV treatment adherence and improve patient outcomes.

ACKNOWLEDGMENTS

The authors are privileged to work closely with many exceptional researchers and treatment providers, so this article benefits from their careful thinking and ideas. Discussions occurred at the March 2006 NIMH/IAPAC International Conference on HIV Treatment Adherence, among other forums. Primary co-sponsorship for the March 2006 conference was provided by the National Institute of Mental Health (NIMH) and the International Association of Physicians in AIDS Care (IAPAC), along with contributions from the National Institute on Drug Abuse (NIDA), the Office of AIDS Research (OAR) at NIH, and other industry support. Thanks to other partnerships in the meeting planning process, interdisciplinary attendees included members of the Association of Nurses in AIDS Care (ANAC), the Society of Infectious Disease Pharmacists (SIDP), and providers funded by the HIV/AIDS Bureau of the Health Resources and Services Administration (HRSA).

NOTE

The views expressed in this commentary do not necessarily represent those of the National Institute of Mental Health or any other agency of the federal government.

REFERENCES

Ahdieh-Grant, L., Silverberg, M. J., Palacio, H., Minkoff, H., Anastos, K., Young, M.A. et al. (2001). Discontinuation of potent antiretroviral therapy: Predictive value of and impact on CD4 cell counts and HIV RNA levels. *AIDS, 15*, 2101-2108.

Ahdieh-Grant, L., Tarwater, P. M., Schneider, M. F., Anastos, K., Cohen, M., Khalsa, A. et al. (2005). Factors and temporal trends associated with highly active antiretroviral therapy discontinuation in the Women's Interagency HIV Study. *Journal of Acquired Immune Deficiency Syndromes, 38,* 500-503.

Ammassari, A., Trotta, M. P., Murri, R., Castelli, F., Narciso, P., Noto, P. et al. (2002). Correlates and predictors of adherence to highly active antiretroviral therapy: Overview of published literature. *Journal of Acquired Immune Deficiency Syndromes, 31,* S123-S127.

Arnsten, J. H., Demas, P. A, Farzadegan, H., Grant, R. W., Gourevitch, M. N., Chang, C. J. et al. (2001). Antiretroviral therapy adherence and viral suppression in HIV-infected drug users: Comparison of self-report and electronic monitoring. *Clinical Infectious Diseases, 33,* 1417-1423.

Bangsberg, D. R. (2006). Less than 95% adherence to nonnucleoside reverse-transcriptase inhibitor therapy can lead to viral suppression. *Clinical Infectious Diseases, 43,* 939-941.

Bangsberg, D. R., Hecht, F. M., Charlebois, E. D., Zolopa, A. R., Holodniy, M., Sheiner, L. et al. (2000). Adherence to protease inhibitors, HIV-1 viral load, and development of drug resistance in an indigent population. *AIDS, 14,* 357-366.

Bangsberg, D. R., Perry, S., Charlebois, E. D., Clark, R. A., Robertson, M., Zolopa, A. R. et al. (2001). Non-adherence to highly active antiretroviral therapy predicts progression to AIDS. *AIDS, 15,* 1181-1183.

Bangsberg, D. R., Simoni, J., Ware, N., & Castro, A. (March, 2006). Developing theoretical models of adherence behavior in resource-limited settings. Paper presented at the 1st International Conference on HIV Treatment Adherence, Jersey City, New Jersey, USA.

Behforouz, H. L., Farmer, P. E., & Mukherjee, J. S. (2004). From directly observed therapy to accompagnateurs: Enhancing AIDS treatment outcomes in Haiti and in Boston. *Clinical Infectious Diseases, 38*(Suppl. 5), S429-S436.

Castilla, J., del Romero, J., Hernando, V., Marincovich, B., Garcia, S., & Rodriguez, C. (2005). Effectiveness of highly active antiretroviral therapy in reducing heterosexual transmission of HIV. *Journal of Acquired Immune Deficiency Syndromes, 40,* 96-101.

Centers for Disease Control and Prevention. (2005). Antiretroviral postexposure prophylaxis after sexual, injection-drug use, or other nonoccupational exposure to HIV in the United States: Recommendations from the U.S. Department of Health and Human Services. *Morbidity and Mortality Weekly Report, 54*(RR-2), 1-19.

Crane, J. T., Kawuma, A., Oyugi, J. H., Byakika, J. T., Moss, A. Bourgois, P. et al. (2006). The price of adherence: Qualitative findings from HIV positive individuals purchasing fixed-dose combination generic HIV antiretroviral therapy in Kampala, Uganda. *AIDS and Behavior, 10,* 437-442.

Farmer, P., Leandre, F., Mukherjee, J. S., Claude, M. S., Nevil, P., Smith-Fawzi, M. C. et al. (2001). Community-based approaches to HIV treatment in resource-poor settings. *Lancet, 358,* 404-409.

Feaster, D., Mitrani, V. B., Prado, G., & Szapocznik, J. (March, 2006). Structural ecosystems therapy for improving HIV medication adherence in African American women. Paper presented at the 1st International Conference on HIV Treatment Adherence, Jersey City, New Jersey, USA.

Fogarty, L., Roter, D., Larson, S., Burke, J., Gillespie, J., & Levy, R. (2002). Patient adherence to HIV medication regimens: A review of published an abstract reports. *Patient Education and Counseling, 46*, 93-108.

Frick, P., Tapia, K., Grant, P., Novotny, M., & Kerzee, J. (2006). The effect of a multidisciplinary program on HAART adherence. *AIDS Patient Care and STDs, 20, 511-524.*

Gandelman, A., & Rietmeijer, C. A. (2004). Translation, adaptation, and synthesis of interventions for persons living with HIV: Lessons from previous HIV prevention interventions. *Journal of Acquired Immune Deficiency Syndromes, 37*(Suppl. 2), S126-S129.

Garcia de Olalla, P., Knobel, H., Carmona, A., Guelar, A., Lopez-Colomes, J. L., & Cayla, J. A. (2002). Impact of adherence and highly active antiretroviral therapy on survival in HIV-infected patients. *Journal of Acquired Immune Deficiency Syndromes, 30, 105-110.*

Gardner, L. I., Metsch, L. R., Anderson-Mahoney, P., Loughlin, A. M., del Rio, C., Strathdee, S. et al. (2005). Efficacy of a brief case management intervention to link recently diagnosed HIV-infected persons to care. *AIDS, 19, 423-431.*

Gebo, K. A., Fleishman, J. A., Conviser, R., Reilly, E. D., Korthuis, P. T., Moore, R. D. et al. (2004). Racial and gender disparities in receipt of highly active antiretroviral therapy persist in a multistate sample of HIV patients in 2001. *Journal of Acquired Immune Deficiency Syndromes, 38*, 96-103.

Giordano, T. P., Visnegarwala, F., White, A. C., Troisi, C. L., Frankowski, R. F. Hartman, C. M. et al. (2005). Patients referred to an urban HIV clinic frequently fail to establish care: Factors predicting failure. *AIDS Care, 17*, 773-783.

Golin, C., Isasi, F., Bontempi, J. B., & Eng, E. (2002). Secret pills: HIV-positive patients' experiences taking antiretroviral therapy in North Carolina. *AIDS Education and Prevention, 14*, 318-329.

Gulick, R. M. (2006). Adherence to antiretroviral therapy: How much is enough? *Clinical Infectious Diseases, 43*, 942-944.

Hogg, R. S., Heath, K., Bangsberg, D., Yip, B., Press, N., O'Shaughnessey, M. V. et al. (2002). Intermittent use of triple-combination therapy is predictive of mortality at baseline and after 1 year of follow-up. *AIDS, 16*, 1051-1058.

Janssen, R. S., Holtgrave, D. R., Valdiserri, R. O., Shepherd, M., Gayle, H. D., & De Cock, K. M. (2001). The Serostatus Approach to Fighting the HIV Epidemic: Prevention strategies for infected individuals. *American Journal of Public Health, 91*, 1019-1024.

Kalichman, S. C., & Rompa, D. (2003). HIV treatment adherence and unprotected sex practices in people receiving antiretroviral therapy. *Sexually Transmitted Infections, 79*, 59-61.

Kayitenkore, K., Bekan, B., Rufagari, J., Marion-Landais, S., Karita, E., & Allen, S. (August, 2006). The impact of ART on HIV transmission among HIV serodiscordant couples [Abstract MOKC101]. Abstract published at the XVI International AIDS Conference, Toronto, Ontario, Canada.

Kidder, D. P., Pals, S. L., Wolitski, R. J., Royal, S., Stall, R., & the Housing and Health Study Team. (August, 2006). HIV medication use, adherence, and disclosure to family members are associated with viral load in homeless or unstably housed HIV positive persons [Abstract TUPE0755]. Abstract published at the XVI International AIDS Conference, Toronto, Ontario, Canada.

King, M. S., Brun, S. C., & Kempf, D. J. (2005). Relationship between adherence and the development of resistance in antiretroviral-naive, HIV-1-infected patients receiving lopinavir/ritonavir or nelfinavir. *Journal of Infectious Diseases, 191*, 2046-2052.

Koenig, S. P., Leandre, F., & Farmer, P. E. (2004). Scaling-up HIV treatment programmes in resource-limited settings: The rural Haiti experience. *AIDS, 18* (Suppl. 3), S21-S25.

Kurth, A. (March, 2006). Antiretroviral adherence assessment. Paper presented at the 1st International Conference on HIV Treatment Adherence, Jersey City, New Jersey, USA.

Liu, A. Y., Grant, R. M., & Buchbinder, S. P. (2006). Preexposure prophylaxis for HIV: Unproven promise and potential pitfalls. *Journal of the American Medical Association, 296*, 863-865.

Maggiolo, F., Ravasio, L., Ripamonti, D., Gregis, G., Quinzan, G., Arici, C. et al. (2005). Similar adherence rates favor different virologic outcomes for patients treated with nonnucleoside analogues or protease inhibitors. *Clinical Infectious Diseases, 40*, 158-163.

Mannheimer, S. B., Botsko, M., Hirschhorn, L. R., Dougherty, J., Celano, S. A., Ciccarone, D. et al. (2006). The CASE adherence index: A novel method for measuring adherence to antiretroviral therapy. Paper presented at the 1st International Conference on HIV Treatment Adherence, Jersey City, New Jersey, USA.

Mitchell, C. G., Freels, S., Creticos, C. M., & Douglas, R. (March, 2006). DAART + : Integrating HIV treatment adherence and prevention. Paper presented at the 1st International Conference on HIV Treatment Adherence, Jersey City, New Jersey, USA.

Mocroft, A., Youle, M., Moore, A., Sabin, C. A., Madge, S., Cozzi Lepri, A. et al. (2001). Reasons for modification and discontinuation of antiretrovirals: Results from a single treatment centre. *AIDS, 15*, 185-194.

Montaner, J. S. G., Hogg, R., Wood, E., Kerr, T., Tyndall, M., Levy, A. R. et al. (2006). The case for expanding access to highly active antiretroviral therapy to curb the growth of the HIV epidemic. *Lancet, 368*, 531-536.

Mugyenyi, P. (March, 2006). Advancing HIV treatment and adherence in Africa. Paper presented at the 1st International Conference on HIV Treatment Adherence, Jersey City, New Jersey, USA.

NIMH/IAPAC International Conference on HIV Treatment Adherence. (2006a). Poster Abstracts, Part 1. *Journal of the International Association of Physicians in AIDS Care, 5*, 11-28.

NIMH/IAPAC International Conference on HIV Treatment Adherence. (2006b). Oral Abstracts. *Journal of the International Association of Physicians in AIDS Care, 5*, 29-39.

NIMH/IAPAC International Conference on HIV Treatment Adherence. (2006c). Poster Abstracts, Part 2. *Journal of the International Association of Physicians in AIDS Care, 5*, 57-82.

Omrani, A. S., & Freedman, A. (2005). Prophylaxis of HIV Infection. *British Medical Bulletin, 73-74*, 93-105.

Palacio, H., Kahn, J. G., Richards, T. A., & Morin, S. F. (2002). Effect of race and/or ethnicity in use of antiretrovirals and prophylaxis for opportunistic infection: A review of the literature. *Public Health Reports, 117*, 233-251.

Paterson, D. L., Swindells, S., Mohr, J., Brester, M., Vergis, E. N., Squier, C. et al. (2000). Adherence to protease inhibitor therapy and outcomes in patients with HIV infection. *Annals of Internal Medicine, 133,* 21-30.

Peretti-Watel, P., Spire, B., Pierret, J., Lert, F., Obadia, Y., & the VESPA Group. (2006). Management of HIV-related stigma and adherence to HAART: Evidence from a large representative sample of outpatients attending French hospitals (ANRS-EN12-VESPA 2003). *AIDS Care, 18,* 254-261.

Reif, S., Whetten, K., Lowe, K., & Ostermann, J. (2006). Association of unmet needs for support services with medication use and adherence among HIV-infected individuals in the southeastern United States. *AIDS Care, 18,* 277-283.

Remien, R. H., Stirratt, M. J., & Dognin, J. S. (March, 2006). Couple-based adherence intervention: How-to. Workshop presented at the 1st International Conference on HIV Treatment Adherence, Jersey City, New Jersey, USA.

Rintamaki, L. S., Davis, T. C., Skripkauskas, S., Bennett, C. L., & Wolf, M. S. (2006). Social stigma concerns and HIV medication adherence. *AIDS Patient Care and STDs, 20,* 359-368.

Sarna, A., Luchters, S., Geibel S., Kaai, S., Munyao, P., Mandaliya, K. et al. (March, 2006). A randomized controlled trial evaluating a directly administered antiretroviral therapy (DAART) intervention to promote adherence to ART in Mombasa, Kenya. Presented at the NIMH/IAPAC 1st International Conference on HIV Treatment Adherence, Newark, New Jersey, USA.

Simoni, J. M., Pearson, C. R., Pantalone, D. W., Crepaz, N., & Marks, G. (March, 2006). State of the ART: Interventions. Paper presented at the 1st International Conference on HIV Treatment Adherence, Jersey City, New Jersey, USA.

Stirratt, M. J., Remien, R. H., Smith, A., Copeland, O. Q., Dolezal, C., Krieger, D., & the SMART Couples Study Team (2006). The role of HIV serostatus disclosure in antiretroviral medication adherence. *AIDS and Behavior, 10,* 483-493.

Stone, V. E. (2004). Optimizing the care of minority patients with HIV/AIDS. *Clinical Infectious Diseases, 38,* 400-404.

Touloumi, G., Pantazis, N., Antoniou, A., Stirnadel, H. A., Walker, S. A., Porter, K. et al. (2006). Highly active antiretroviral therapy interruption: Predictors and virologic and immunologic consequences. *Journal of Acquired Immune Deficiency Syndromes, 42,* 554-561.

Valdiserri, R. O. (2004). International scale-up for antiretroviral treatment: Where does prevention fit? *Journal of Acquired Immune Deficiency Syndromes, 37* (Suppl. 2), S138-S141.

Velasco-Hernandez, J. X., Gershengorn, H. B., & Blower, S. M. (2002). Could widespread use of combination antiretroviral therapy eradicate HIV epidemics? *Lancet Infectious Diseases, 2,* 487-493.

Weiser, S., Wolfe, W., Bangsberg, D., Thior, I., Gilbert, P., Makhema, J. et al. (2003). Barriers to antiretroviral adherence for patients living with HIV infection and AIDS in Botswana. *Journal of Acquired Immune Deficiency Syndromes, 34,* 281-288.

Youle, M., & Wainberg, M. A. (2003). Pre-exposure chemoprophylaxis (PREP) as an HIV prevention strategy. *Journal of the International Association of Physicians in AIDS Care, 2,* 102-105.

doi:10.1300/J187v06n01_02

Psychosocial Predictors of Adherence to Highly Active Antiretroviral Therapy: Practical Implications

Valerie A. Gruber, PhD, MPH
James L. Sorensen, PhD
Nancy A. Haug, PhD

SUMMARY. This article reviews studies of psychosocial predictors of Highly Active Antiretroviral Therapy (HAART) among HIV positive clients. Unstable housing and lack of HIV-specific social support predicted low HAART adherence in the studies where they were tested. The

---

Valerie A. Gruber, PhD, MPH, is an Associate Clinical Professor at the Department of Psychiatry, University of California San Francisco, and serves as Attending Psychologist at San Francisco General Hospital.

James L. Sorensen, PhD, is a Professor at the Department of Psychiatry, University of California San Francisco, and serves as Attending Psychologist at San Francisco General Hospital.

Nancy A. Haug, PhD, is an Assistant Adjunct Professor at the Department of Psychiatry, University of California San Francisco, and serves as Attending Psychologist at San Francisco General Hospital.

Address correspondence to: Valerie Gruber, PhD, MPH, Associate Clinical Professor, Department of Psychiatry at the University of California San Francisco, 3180 18th Street, Suite 202, San Francisco, CA 94110 (E-mail: Valerie.Gruber@sfdph.org).

Support for this project was provided by the National Institute on Drug Abuse grant P50 DA09253, and the California-Arizona Clinical Trials Network Research Node cooperative agreement U10DA15815.

[Haworth co-indexing entry note]: "Psychosocial Predictors of Adherence to Highly Active Antiretroviral Therapy: Practical Implications." Gruber, Valerie A., James L. Sorensen, and Nancy A. Haug. Co-published simultaneously in *the Journal of HIV/AIDS & Social Services* (The Haworth Press, Inc.) Vol. 6, No. 1/2, 2007, pp. 23-37; and: *HIV Treatment Adherence: Challenges for Social Services* (ed: Lana Sue Ka'opua and Nathan L. Linsk) The Haworth Press, Inc., 2007, pp. 23-37. Single or multiple copies of this article are available for a fee from The Haworth Document Delivery Service [1-800-HAWORTH, 9:00 a.m. - 5:00 p.m. (EST). E-mail address: docdelivery@haworthpress.com].

Available online at http://jhaso.haworthpress.com
© 2007 by The Haworth Press, Inc. All rights reserved.
doi: 10.1300/J187v06n01_03

most consistent predictor of adherence problems across all populations and measures was active substance use, particularly cocaine use. Younger age and less than high school education were not consistently predictive. Depression predicted adherence problems measured by self-report but not by electronic monitoring. Supplementing the adherence support efforts by physicians, nurses, and pharmacists, clinicians in a range of disciplines and settings can assess and intervene on psychosocial risk factors and thereby reduce adherence problems regardless of their level of knowledge about HIV medications. doi:10.1300/J187v06n01_03 *[Article copies available for a fee from The Haworth Document Delivery Service: 1-800-HAWORTH. E-mail address: <docdelivery@haworthpress.com> Website: <http://www.HaworthPress.com> © 2007 by The Haworth Press, Inc. All rights reserved.]*

KEYWORDS. Adherence, compliance, Highly Active Antiretroviral Therapy, psychosocial

INTRODUCTION

Effective treatment of HIV and AIDS requires adherence to complex regimens of Highly Active Antiretroviral Therapy (HAART). In a study of homeless and marginally housed people with HIV, "each 10% difference in adherence was associated with a 28% reduction in risk of progression to AIDS" (Bangsberg, Perry et al., 2001, p. 118). The best assurance against developing drug resistant virus and for keeping viral load low is near-perfect adherence, i.e., taking 95% of doses or more (Bangsberg, Moss, & Deeks, 2004; Gathe, 2003).

HAART generally involves three or more medications that each need to be taken as directed several times a day, and with or without food. The demanding dosing schedule, in combination with side effects, makes it unusually difficult to take these medications exactly as prescribed (Chesney, 2000). Barriers to adherence fall into four groups: (1) medication variables (e.g., dosing complexity, side effects); (2) patient variables (psychosocial and clinical characteristics); (3) patient-health-care provider relationship variables; and (4) system of care variables (Chesney, 2000). This review focuses on the second category, specifically, psychosocial risk factors for adherence problems.

This review is relevant to health care providers, in that patients with psychosocial risk factors for HAART adherence problems need to be identified and referred to psychosocial services. Moreover, this review is relevant to clinicians from a variety of disciplines who provide these psychosocial services either within medical settings or in other settings. These settings include, but are not limited to mental health, substance abuse, case management, housing, and social service programs. If psychosocial risk factors for adherence problems (category 2 above) can be addressed by staff with the skills and resources to change them, then clients will be more able to benefit from the medication adherence tools provided by medical clinics and pharmacies (categories 1, 3, and 4).

METHODS

We reviewed the clinical research literature to determine what knowledge base existed on problems in HAART adherence among HIV positive patients. We examined the PubMed and PsycINFO databases for prospective studies of adults in peer reviewed journals, using the key words (1) Adherence or Compliance, and (2) HAART. This yielded four studies (Carrieri et al., 2003; Levine et al., 2005; Spire et al., 2002; Weaver et al., 2005).

To identify additional studies of HAART, we substituted the term with "antiretroviral" and searched for publications from 1998-2005. This yielded ten additional studies of HAART adherence (Godin, Cote, Naccache, Lambert, & Trottier, 2005; Golin et al., 2002; Hinkin et al., 2004; Howard et al., 2002; Matthews et al., 2002; Samet, Horton, Meli, Freedberg, & Palepu, 2004; Wagner, 2002), including three with methadone maintenance clients (Avants, Margolin, Warburton, Hawkins, & Shi, 2001; Arnsten et al., 2002; Berg et al., 2004).

Supplementing the PubMed/PsycINFO search, a recent literature review (Uldall, Palmer, Whetten, & Mellins, 2004) mentioned several conference proceedings and federally funded studies in progress. Follow up on these yielded three additional published studies (Bouhnik et al., 2002; Halkitis, Kutnik, & Slater, 2005; Mellins, Kang, Leu, Havens, & Chesney, 2003).

In the seventeen prospective studies identified, the largest groups of people with HIV were adequately represented. In the studies conducted in the U.S., 42%-93% of participants were people of color. In most studies, 20% or more of participants were women. In three of the studies with fewer women, a majority of participants were men who had sex with men (Halkitis et al., 2005; Matthews et al., 2002; Wagner, 2002). We included the three studies conducted in methadone maintenance clinics. Despite the frequency of psychosocial problems, approximately half of methadone maintenance clients achieve 95% adherence, equivalent to other HIV populations studied (Palmer, Salcedo, Miller, Winiarski, & Arno, 2003; Stein et al., 2000).

The seventeen prospective studies identified were all of high quality. All studies used multivariate analysis to control for confounding between variables. Ten of the studies measured adherence electronically using pill bottles with microchips embedded in the caps. Of these ten, five used only electronic adherence measures (Arnsten et al., 2002; Berg et al., 2004; Hinkin et al., 2004; Howard et al., 2002; Levine et al., 2005); three combined electronic monitoring and self-report into composite adherence measures (Golin et al., 2002; Halkitis et al., 2005; Weaver et al., 2005); and two analyzed electronically monitored and self-reported adherence separately, with self-report measures covering the prior three days (Wagner, 2002) or the prior 30 days (Matthews et al., 2002). Seven of the studies measured adherence by self-report only (Avants et al., 2001; Bouhnik et al., 2002; Carrieri et al., 2003; Godin et al., 2005; Mellins et al., 2003; Samet et al., 2004; Spire et al., 2002). All of these asked participants about the past two to seven days, a short period that is less prone to recall problems than longer reporting periods.

FINDINGS

Variables Related to HAART Adherence

Two variables were consistently predictive in multivariate analyses. Stable housing consistently predicted better HAART medication adherence, and stimulant use consistently predicted poorer HAART medication adherence.

Stable housing predicted HAART adherence in the one electronic monitoring study where it was tested (Table 1). In this study, methadone maintenance clients with permanent housing took 75% of HAART medication doses, versus 42% among those without long-term housing. In multivariate analysis adjusting for other variables, having long-term housing led to an average of 16 more doses taken on time over a six month period (Berg et al., 2004, p. 1114). Likewise, in a study measuring adherence by self-report, stable housing was predictive in multivariate analyses (Spire et al., 2002, p. 1490).

TABLE 1. Stable Housing

Study	Sample	Effect Found
Studies of Electronically Monitored Adherence		
Berg et al. '04	113 MM clients, New York	75% vs. 42% of doses ***
Studies of Self-Reported Adherence		
Spire et al. '02	445 HIV clinic patients, France	OR = 2.76 (1.3-5.85)

Note. MM = methadone maintenance.
OR = multivariate odds ratio (with 95% confidence interval).
If 95% confidence interval excludes 1.0, then $p < .05$.
NS is defined as $p > .05$. $^* p < .05$. $^{**} p < .01$. $^{***} p < .005$.

HIV specific social support predicted HAART adherence when controlling for other variables in the one study where it was tested. Methadone maintenance clients who participated in an HIV support group had 84% on time medication cap openings, in contrast to 54% among those who did not (Berg et al., 2004, p. 1114). In contrast to the effect found for HIV specific social support, *general social support* was not predictive in the two electronic monitoring studies testing it (Golin et al., 2002; Weaver et al., 2005), and barely reached significance in predicting adherence, with an Odds Ratio (OR) of 1.06 and a 95% confidence interval of 1.02-1.11, in one of the two self-report studies testing it (Samet et al., 2004, p. 574). Similarly, relationship status was not predictive in any of the five electronic monitoring studies testing it (Arnsten et al., 2002; Berg et al., 2004; Golin et al., 2002; Halkitis et al., 2005; Matthews et al., 2002); it was only predictive in the three self-report studies testing it (Carrieri et al., 2003; Godin et al., 2005; Matthews et al., 2002).

Cocaine use predicted HAART adherence problems in multivariate analyses in all but one small study (Avants et al., 2001; N = 42). *Amphetamine use* predicted electronically monitored adherence problems in the one study where it was tested (Matthews et al., 2002). In contrast to stimulants, heroin and alcohol use had smaller and less consistent effects (Tables 2 and 3). Heroin use predicted lower adherence among women (40% versus 70% of doses) but not men in one study (Berg et al., 2004, p. 1114), and was not predictive in two studies that did not stratify heroin use by gender (Arnsten et al., 2002; Avants et al., 2001). In one study adherence was unrelated to a combined substance use disorder category that had only 23 participants in it (Wagner, 2002).

TABLE 2. Substance Use in Studies of Electronically Monitored Adherence

Study	Sample	Effect Found
Mathews et al. '02	164 HIV clinic patients	*Amphetamine:* OR = .2 (.1-.6) *Alcohol:* NS
Howard et al. '02	161 women in 4 U.S. cities	*Cocaine or heroin:* 34% vs. 57% of doses *** *Alcohol:* 43% vs. 56% of doses *
Golin et al. '02	140 public HIV clinic patients	*Drugs:* 59% vs. 72% adherent * *Alcohol:* 66% vs. 74% adherent **
Arnsten et al. '02	85 MM clients, New York	*Cocaine:* 27% vs. 68% of doses * *Heroin, alcohol:* both NS
Berg et al. '04	113 MM clients, New York	*Cocaine:* 29% vs. 72% of doses ** *Heroin, alcohol:* both NS
Hinkin et al. '04	148 Los Angeles residents	*Cocaine:* 7% v 35% good adherers * *Alcohol:* NS
Halkitis et al. '05	300 MSM, New York	*Cocaine:* 83% vs. 91% of doses **
Wagner '02	173 Los Angeles residents	*Substance abuse or dependence:* NS
Levine et al. '05	222 Los Angeles residents	*Substance abuse or dependence:* Chi-sq. = 17.0 ***

Note. MM = methadone maintenance. MSM = men who have sex with men.
OR = multivariate odds ratio (with 95% confidence interval).
If 95% confidence interval excludes 1.0, then $p < .05$.
NS is defined as $p > .05$.   * $p < .05$.   ** $p < .01$.   *** $p < .005$.

TABLE 3. Substance Use in Studies of Self-reported Adherence

Study	Sample	Effect Found
Avants et. al. '01	42 MM clients, Boston	*Cocaine, opiate use:* both NS
Mathews et al. '02	164 HIV clinic patients	*Cocaine:* OR = .03 (.00-.44) *Alcohol:* NS
Carrieri et al. '03	96 infected by IDU, France	*Current IDU:* OR = 3.3 (1.0-10.3)
Spire et al. '02	445 HIV clinic patients, France	*One drink or less/day:* OR = 1.7 (1.03-2.8)
Bouhnik et al. '02	210 ex-IDUs, not in MM, France	Amount of *alcohol:* NS
Samet et al. '04	267 past alcohol abusers, Boston	*Not drinking:* OR = 3.6 (2.0-4.5)
Wagner '02	173 Los Angeles residents	*Substance abuse or dependence:* NS
Mellins et al. '03	93 female HIV clinic patients	*Substance abuse or dependence:* OR (missed pills) = 7.32 (1.5-34.4)
Halkitis et al. '05	300 MSM, New York	*Cocaine:* 92% vs. 96% of doses *

Note. IDU = injection drug use. MM = methadone maintenance. MSM = men who have sex with men.
OR = multivariate odds ratio (with 95% confidence interval).
If 95% confidence interval excludes 1.0, then $p < .05$.
NS is defined as $p > .05$.   * $p < .05$.   ** $p < .01$.   *** $p < .005$.

Variables Mostly Unrelated to HAART Adherence

Three variables were sometimes predictive, but were mostly not associated with HAART adherence. These included age, education, and depression.

Older age predicted slightly better electronically monitored HAART adherence in some studies (Howard et al., 2002; Levine et al., 2005; Weaver et al., 2005), but was unrelated in five others (Berg et al., 2004; Golin et al., 2002; Halkitis et al., 2005; Matthews et al., 2002; Wagner, 2002). Likewise, age predicted better self-reported adherence in two studies (Mellins et al., 2003; Spire et al., 2002), but was unrelated in five others (Avants et al., 2001; Bouhnik et al., 2002; Matthews et al., 2002; Samet et al., 2004; Wagner, 2002).

One electronic monitoring study suggested a nonlinear relationship. Among people less than 50 years old, only 26% took 95% of their doses or more, in contrast to 53% of people age 50 or above; the odds ratio was 3.1 (1.4-6.76) (Hinkin et al., 2004, p. S22). The connection between younger age and adherence problems may relate in part to number of children in the household, which predicted lower self-reported adherence in the two studies where it was tested (Mellins et al., 2003; Wagner, 2002).

Education, controlling for other variables, predicted slightly higher HAART adherence in an electronic monitoring study where education was classified as less than high school, or high school or above (Golin et al., 2002), and in a self-report study where education ranged from grades 8-17 (Avants et al., 2001). However, number of years of education was unrelated to adherence problems in all other studies where it was tested (Howard et al., 2002; Levine et al., 2005; Spire et al., 2002; Wagner, 2002; Weaver et al., 2005).

Depression was unrelated to electronically monitored HAART adherence in all six studies where it was tested (Arnsten et al., 2002; Berg et al., 2004; Halkitis et al., 2005; Levine et al., 2005; Matthews et al., 2002; Wagner, 2002). In contrast, depression did predict self-reported adherence problems in multivariate analyses in seven studies where it was tested (Avants et al., 2001; Bouhnik et al., 2002; Carrieri et al., 2003; Mellins et al., 2003; Samet et al., 2004; Spire et al., 2002; Wagner, 2002). Thus although depressed people opened their medication bottles on time as much as others, they were more likely to recall and admit adherence problems than non-depressed people.

DISCUSSION

Unstable housing and cocaine use are the most consistent psychosocial predictors of HAART adherence problems. Although amphetamine use was tested in only one study, it is a stimulant similar to cocaine, and like cocaine it is often used in a binge pattern; therefore, similar effects on adherence can be expected.

Although social support is important to many aspects of a person's quality of life, the studies reviewed here indicate that helping clients obtain social support will not do much for their adherence to HAART. This is remarkable because social support has been related to adherence problems in prior studies that used self-report measures and cross-sectional designs. In contrast to general social support, HIV specific support groups appears to improve adherence; however, only one study tested this (Berg et al., 2004).

Depression predicted adherence problems when measured by self-report but not when assessed using electronic monitoring. Although depression has been a consistent predictor of adherence problems in medical care (Chesney, 2000), it did not predict electronically monitored adherence in any of the six prospective studies of HAART medication adherence. This occurred despite sufficient variability in depression in most of these studies, and regardless of whether depression was measured by diagnostic interview or by Beck Depression Inventory scores. In each of these studies, depressed people opened their medication bottles on time as much as others. It could be that people suffering from depression have difficulty completing medication ingestion (e.g., coordinating the medications with meals, swallowing large pills). Because depression causes people to think and talk more about problems, it is also possible that depressed people recall adherence problems more or admit to them more freely than others do.

Younger age, and less than high school education were related to HAART adherence problems in some studies but unrelated in others. Consistent with research involving other adherence requirements and other diseases, difficulties with HAART medication adherence impact all age and economic groups.

By way of limitations, the studies used a variety of adherence measures, making cross-study comparisons difficult. In particular, self-report overestimates adherence (Liu et al., 2001). An additional limitation is that some studies had few participants in some groups, which limited the sensitivity of statistical comparisons. A next step might be to conduct a meta-analysis; this method combines studies for increased statistical power, while weighting them by methodological quality. This might clarify the effects of the variables where findings are inconsistent. Even without meta-analysis, however, the evidence is substantial that housing instability and stimulant use interfere with adherence to HAART medications.

PRACTICAL IMPLICATIONS

Identifying Clients Who Need Adherence Support and Psychosocial Interventions

Health care providers in busy medical clinics must often rely on patients' self-reported adherence supplemented by their own estimates, both of which overestimate adherence (Bangsberg, Hecht et al., 2001; Liu et al., 2001). To identify additional patients with adherence problems, it can be helpful to screen for risk factors for HAART adherence problems, as described below. Individuals who screen in with risk factors can receive additional adherence supports such as reminder systems, and can be referred to services addressing the risk factors themselves. In addition, psychiatric, substance abuse, or social service staff often conduct more extensive psychosocial assessments and can thus identify additional individuals who have psychosocial risk factors for adherence problems; they can intervene on the risk factors and inform patients' health care providers of their risk for adherence problems.

In some settings, people are reluctant to disclose the major psychosocial risk factors, unstable housing and stimulant use. For example, in general medical clinics serving employees and other insured individuals, patients may withhold substance use information so that it cannot inadvertently be revealed to employers or insurance companies. To screen most broadly for possible HAART adherence risk without asking people to disclose sensitive information, one can use a brief indicator reflective of both established and less established risk factors. One such tool is the 4-item version of the Perceived Stress Scale (French et al., 2005). It asks four simple questions: "In the past month, how often have you felt (a) unable to control the important things in your life, (b) confident in your ability to handle their personal problems, (c) that things were going your way, and (d) that difficulties were piling up so high that you could not handle them." Each question is rated "never/rarely, sometimes, often, or mostly/always" (p. 591). This measure does not require clients to disclose details they may prefer to keep private. Despite its simplicity and generality, people in the top quartile are more likely to have adherence problems than those in the bottom quartile; with an OR of 2.16 (1.15-4.07) when adjusted for other predictors (French et al., 2005, p. 594).

In settings where people tend to disclose unstable housing and substance use more freely, such as in HIV specialty clinics serving uninsured people, brief screens for unstable housing and substance use can quickly identify individuals with the most certain risk for HAART adherence problems. In many medical clinics, this simply involves using information that is already collected. Patient check-in procedures routinely include address updates, and medical history forms routinely inquire about substance use. However, brief screenings without detailed prompts can easily miss some problems. If the person gives an address, they appear to have a stable residence but may in fact be there only temporarily or intermittently. Similarly, a single broad question about drug use can easily be evaded with a terse answer of "none."

The most certain way to identify unstable housing and stimulant use is during comprehensive psychosocial needs assessments. Case managers, mental health providers, substance abuse treatment providers, or other social services staff usually conduct these. However, psychosocial assessment tools tend to focus on the issues addressed by the particular setting and do not necessarily assess both housing and stimulant use. For example, the Addiction Severity Index (McLellan et al., 1992), a structured interview used in many addiction treatment programs, assesses use of a variety of drugs and alcohol and the negative effects thereof, but with respect to housing instability only asks for address and duration at that address. Thus clinicians need to follow up with additional probes, such as whether they have a home, and if not how long they have been homeless. Programs and treatment systems that have the capacity to modify the assessment instruments they use may want to consider adding these or similar questions or prompts, modified as appropriate to local conditions and cultural considerations (e.g., Katrina Hurricane dislocation).

Interventions for Psychosocial Risk Factors

It can be immensely helpful to simply acknowledge with clients that HAART is one of the most demanding medication regimens, and that adherence problems are common. This allows clients to feel less shame and speak more openly about adherence problems with all those providing care associated with improving health outcomes be they health care, mental health, substance abuse treatment, or social service providers. Once they are comfortable with the idea of speaking to others about HIV and adherence issues, they can be referred to an HIV support group to help them cope with adherence and other HIV related challenges.

The connection between housing instability and medication adherence problems is usually painfully obvious to those affected by it. For example, leaving home on short notice to avoid domestic violence, or staying with different friends for a few days at a time each run the risk of inadvertently leaving medications behind. The previously used pharmacy may be difficult to get to after moving, requiring that all the prescriptions and refills be reestablished with a new pharmacy. Because of the chronic shortage of affordable housing in most areas, helping clients obtain stable housing often requires extensive time and effort by social service staff knowledgeable about local housing options and entry criteria.

For substance use, the connection to medication adherence needs to be introduced to clients without eliciting feelings of shame about their use. If they approach it without judgment, clinical staff in any setting can help clients recognize how their adherence plummets during use of stimulants or other substances, and using a motivational interviewing approach (Miller & Rollnick, 2002; Wagner & Conners, 2005) can help them develop realistic plans for changing their drug use. For some, this may mean starting low-threshold outpatient treatment. For others it may mean obtaining or switching to more intensive or targeted type of drug treatment (e.g., if unable to stop or reduce use of stimulants in outpatient treatment, entering stimulant specific intensive outpatient treatment using a cognitive-behavioral approach).

Each of the psychosocial predictors of HAART adherence problems is amenable to intervention by mental health, substance abuse service, and/or social service providers. These are issues that these clinicians routinely target in their work with clients. Whenever they address one or more of these psychosocial variables, they are helping with medication adherence, even without additional demands on their time, and even without detailed knowledge of HIV medications. Because the problems often aggravate each other (e.g., housing instability worsened by heavy substance use), clinicians with expertise in certain areas need to collaborate with clinicians with expertise in other areas. For example, a heavy substance user needing supportive housing who has "burned their bridges" with the local supportive housing programs may need both specialized addiction treatment (such as methadone maintenance) and a case manager with excellent working relationships with the supportive housing programs.

Systems Development

To facilitate the frequent collaborations between staff with different areas of expertise, many services are being co-located with each other, in settings clients return to repeatedly. One approach is to add psychosocial services to HIV medical clinics. Many HIV medical clinics have added onsite case management, psychiatric, and substance abuse service providers. Another approach is to locate adherence supports and psychosocial services in substance abuse treatment programs. Adherence support by physicians, nurses, and pharmacists can be made more accessible by locating them in or adjacent to drug treatment programs that clients attend weekly or more often, such as outpatient programs or methadone clinics (Batki & Selwyn, 2002; Selwyn et al., 1989).

Likewise, there are frequent opportunities for substance abuse, mental health, and case management staff located at drug treatment programs to address psychosocial risk factors for adherence problems. Because cocaine and methamphetamine use have the most impact on medication adherence, effective treatment for these needs to be made available in every community. Although no medications have yet been found to have a sizeable effect, randomized studies have demonstrated the effectiveness of cognitive-behavioral treatment (e.g., Carroll et al., 1994; Rawson et al., 2004) and contingency management rewarding drug-free urine tests (e.g., Petry et al., 2005; Shoptaw et al., 2006).

CONCLUSION

Helping clients take their HAART medications consistently as prescribed can reduce progression of HIV disease, thereby improving quality of life for both clients and their loved ones. Clinicians in a variety of settings can identify the psychosocial factors that act as barriers to medication adherence. Our review indicates that two of the most salient barriers are housing instability and continued use of substances, especially stimulants. These are also two of the most challenging psychosocial problems to change. The clinician, rather than going it alone, will be well advised to build strong collaborations with colleagues in other disciplines, to increase the likelihood of helping clients make gains in stabilizing their situations, so they can improve their HIV medication adherence, thus improving their overall health.

REFERENCES

* Arnsten, J. H., Demas, P. A., Grant, R. W., Gourevitch, M. N., Farzadegan, H., Howard, A. A. et al. (2002). Impact of active drug use on antiretroviral therapy adherence and viral suppression in HIV-infected drug users. *Journal of General Internal Medicine, 17*(5), 377-81, doi:10.1046/j.1525-1497.2002.10644.x.

* Avants, S. K., Margolin, A., Warburton, L. A., Hawkins, K. A., & Shi, J. (2001). Predictors of nonadherence to HIV-related medication regimens during methadone stabilization. *American Journal of Addictions, 10*(1), 69-78, doi:10.1080/105504901750160501.

Bangsberg, D. R., Moss, A. R., & Deeks, S. G. (2004). Paradoxes of adherence and drug resistance to HIV antiretroviral therapy. *Journal of Antimicrobial Chemotherapy, 53*, 696-699, doi:10.1093/jac/dkh162.

Bangsberg, D. R., Hecht, F. M., Clague, H., Charlebois, E. D., Ciccarone, D., Chesney, M. et al. (2001). Provider assessment of adherence to HIV antiretroviral therapy. *Journal of Acquired Immune Deficiency Syndrome, 26*(5), 435-42.

Bangsberg, D. R., Perry, S., Charlebois, E. D., Clark, R. A., Robertson, M., Zalopa, A. R. et al. (2001). Non-adherence to highly active antiretroviral therapy predicts progression to AIDS. *AIDS, 15*(9), 1181-3, doi:10.1097/00002030-200106150-00015.

Batki, S. L., & Selwyn, P. A. (2002). *Substance abuse treatment for persons with HIV/AIDS: Treatment improvement protocol (TIP) series: 37.* Rockville, MD: U.S. Department of Health and Human Services, Public Health Service, Substance Abuse and Mental Health Services Administration, Center for Substance Abuse Treatment. http://www.kap.samhsa.gov/products/manuals/tips/numerical.htm.

* Berg, K. M., Demas, P. A., Howard, A. A., Schoenbaum, E. E., Gourevitch, M. N., & Arnsten, J. H. (2004). Gender differences in factors associated with adherence to antiretroviral therapy. *Journal of General Internal Medicine, 19*(11), 1111-7, doi: 10.1111/j.1525-1497.2004.30445.x.

* Bouhnik, A. D., Chesney, M., Carrieri, P., Gallais, H., Moreau, J., Moatti, J. P. et al. (2002). Nonadherence among HIV-infected injecting drug users: The impact of social instability. *Journal of Acquired Immune Deficiency Syndrome, 31*(Suppl. 3), S149-53.

* Carrieri, M. P., Chesney, M. A., Spire, B., Loundou, A., Sobel, A., Lepeu, G. et al. (2003). Failure to maintain adherence to HAART in a cohort of French HIV-positive injecting drug users. *International Journal of Behavioral Medicine, 10*(1), 1-14, doi:10.1207/S15327558IJBM1001_01.

Carroll, K. M., Rounsaville, B. J., Nich, C., Gordon, L. T., Wirtz, P. W., & Gawin, F. (1994). One-year follow-up of psychotherapy and pharmacotherapy for cocaine dependence. Delayed emergence of psychotherapy effects. *Archives of General Psychiatry, 51*(12), 989-997.

Chesney, M. A. (2000). Factors affecting adherence to antiretroviral therapy. *Clinical Infectious Diseases, 30*(Suppl. 2), S171-6, doi:10.1086/313849.

French, T., Weiss, L., Waters, M., Tesoriero, J., Finkelstein, R., & Agins, B. (2005). Correlation of a brief perceived stress measure with nonadherence to antiretroviral therapy over time. *Journal of Acquired Immune Deficiency Syndrome, 38*(5), 590-596, doi:10.1097/01.qai.0000135960.88543.8d.

Gathe, J. (2003). Adherence and potency with antiretroviral therapy: A combination for success. *Journal of Acquired Immune Deficiency Syndrome, 34*(Suppl. 2), S118-S122.

* Godin, G., Cote, J., Naccache, H., Lambert, L. D., & Trottier, S. (2005). Prediction of adherence to antiretroviral therapy: A one-year longitudinal study. *AIDS Care, 17*(4), 493-504.

* Golin, C. E., Liu, H., Hays, R. D., Miller, L. G., Beck, C. K., Ickovics, J. et al. (2002). A prospective study of predictors of adherence to combination antiretroviral medication. *Journal of General Internal Medicine, 17*(10), 756-65, doi:10.1046/j.1525-1497.2002.11214.x.

* Halkitis, P. N., Kutnik, A. H., & Slater, S. (2005). The social realities of adherence to protease inhibitor regimens: Substance use, health care, and psychological states. *Health Psychology, 10*(4), 545-58, doi:10.1177/1359105305053422.

* Hinkin, C. H., Hardy, D. J., Mason, K. I., Castellon, S. A., Durvasula, R. S., Lam, M. N. et al. (2004). Medication adherence in HIV-infected adults: Effect of patient age, cognitive status, and substance abuse. *AIDS, 18*(Suppl. 1): S19-S25, doi:10.1097/00002030-200401001-00004.

* Howard, A. A., Arnsten, J. H., Lo, Y., Vlahov, D., Rich, J. D., Schuman, P. et al. (2002). A prospective study of adherence and viral load in a large multi-center cohort of HIV-infected women. *AIDS, 16*(16), 2175-82, doi:10.1097/00002030-200211080-00010.

* Levine, A. J., Hinkin, C. H., Castellon, S. A., Mason, K. I., Lam, M. N., Perkins, A. et al. (2005). Variations in patterns of highly active antiretroviral therapy (HAART) adherence. *AIDS and Behavior, 9*(3), 355-362. doi; 0.1007/s10461-005-9009-y.

Liu, H., Golin, C., Miller, L., Hays, R., Beck, K., Sanandaji, S. et al. (2001). A comparison study of multiple measures of adherence to HIV protease inhibitors. *Annals of Internal Medicine,134*, 968-77.

* Mathews, W. C., Mar-Tang, M., Ballard, C., Colwell, B., Abulhosn, K., Noonan, C. et al. (2002). Prevalence, predictors, and outcomes of early adherence after starting or changing antiretroviral therapy. *AIDS Patient Care and STDs, 16*(4), 167-72, doi:10.1089/10872910252930867.

McLellan, A. T., Kushner, H., Metzger, D., Peters, R., Smith, I., Grissom, G. et al. (1992). The fifth edition of the addiction severity index. *Journal of Substance Abuse Treatment, 9*(3), 199-213, doi:10.1016/0740-5472(92)90062-S.

* Mellins, C. A., Kang, E., Leu, C. S., Havens, J. F., & Chesney, M. A. (2003). Longitudinal study of mental health and psychosocial predictors of medical treatment adherence in mothers living with HIV disease. *AIDS Patient Care and STDs, 17*(8), 407-16, doi:10.1089/108729103322277420.

Miller, W. R., & Rollnick, S. (2002). Motivational interviewing: Preparing people for change (2nd Ed.). New York: Guilford Press. www.motivationalinterview.org.

Palmer, N. B. Salcedo, J., Miller, A. L., Winiarski, M., & Arno, P. (2003). Psychiatric and social barriers to HIV medication adherence in a triply diagnosed methadone population. *AIDS Patient Care and STDs, 17*(12), 635-44, doi:10.1089/108729-103771928690.

Petry, N. M., Peirce, J. M., Stizer, M. L., Blaine, J., Roll, J. M., Cohen, A. et al. (2005). Effect of prize-based incentives on outcomes in stimulant abusers in outpatient psychosocial treatment programs: A national drug abuse treatment clinical trials network study. *Archives of General Psychiatry, 62*(10), 1148-1156. doi: 10.1001/archpsyc.62.10.1148.

Rawson, R. A., Marinelli-Casey, P., Anglin, M. D., Dickow, A., Frazier, Y., Gallagher, C. et al. (2004). A multi-site comparison of psychosocial approaches for the treatment of methamphetamine dependence. *Addiction, 99*(6),708-717. doi:10.1111/j.1360-0443.2004.00707.x.

Samet, J. H., Horton, N. J., Meli, S., Freedberg, K. A., & Palepu, A. (2004). Alcohol consumption and antiretroviral adherence among HIV infected persons with alcohol problems. *Alcoholism: Clinical and Experimental Research, 28*(4), 572-7.

Selwyn, P. A., Feingold, A. R., Iezza, A., Satyadeo, M., Colley, J., Torres, R. et al. (1989). Primary care for patients with human immunodeficiency virus (HIV) infection in a methadone maintenance treatment program. *Annals of Internal Medicine, 111*(9), 761-3.

Shoptaw, S., Huber, A., Peck, J., Yang, X., Liu, J., Dang, J. et al. (2006, in press). Randomized, placebo-controlled trial of sertraline and contingency management for the treatment of methamphetamine dependence. *Drug and Alcohol Dependence,* doi: 10.1016/j.drugalcdep.2006.03.005.

* Spire, B., Duran, S., Souville, M., Leport, C., Raffi, F., Moatti, J. P. et al. (2002). Adherence to HAART in HIV infected patients: From a predictive to a dynamic approach. *Social Science and Medicine, 54*(10), 1481-96, doi:10.1016/S0277-9536(01)00125-3.

Stein, M. D., Rich, J. D., Maksad, J., Chen, M. H., Hu, P., Sobota, M. et al. (2000). Adherence to antiretroviral therapy among HIV-infected methadone patients: Effect of ongoing illicit drug use. *American Journal of Drug and Alcohol Abuse, 26*(2), 195-205, doi:10.1081/ADA-100100600.

Uldall, K. K., Palmer, N. B., Whetten, K., & Mellins, C. (2004). Adherence in people living with HIV/AIDS, mental illness, and chemical dependency: A review of the literature. *AIDS Care, 16*(Suppl. 1), S71-S96, doi:10.1080/09540120412331315277.

* Wagner, G. J. (2002). Predictors of antiretroviral adherence as measured by self-report, electronic monitoring, and medication diaries. *AIDS Patient Care and STDs, 16*(12), 599-608, doi:10.1089/108729102761882134.

Wagner, C., & Conners, W. (2005). MI bibliography (1983-2005). Retrieved on June 2, 2006 from the Motivational Interviewing Page sponsored by the Mid-Atlantic Addiction Technology Transfer Center, In cooperartion with the Motivation Interviewing Network of Trainers (MINT), William R. Miller, PhD, and Stephen Rollinick, PhD. at http://www.motivationalinterview.org/library/biblio.html.

* Weaver, K. E., Llabre, M. M., Duran, R. E., Antoni, M. H., Ironson, G., Penedo, F. J. et al. (2005). A stress and coping model of medication adherence and viral load in HIV positive men and women on highly active antiretroviral therapy (HAART). *Health Psychology, 24*(4), 385-92, doi:10.1037/0278-6133.24.4.385.

References marked with an asterisk (*) indicate studies included in the review.

doi:10.1300/J187v06n01_03

The Relationship Between Type and Quality of Social Support and HIV Medication Adherence

Marie M. Hamilton, MA, MPH
Lisa A. Razzano, PhD
Nicole B. Martin, MS, LCPC

SUMMARY. In the last 10 years HIV has become a disease that can be effectively managed using antiretroviral medications. However, many

Marie M. Hamilton, MA, MPH, is Project Manager; Lisa A. Razzano, PhD, is Associate Professor of Psychiatry and Director of Training & Education Programs; and Nicole B. Martin, MS, LCPC, is Medication Specialist and Research Assistant; all are at the University of Illinois at Chicago, Center on Mental Health Services Research & Policy, Department of Psychiatry.

Address correspondence to: Marie M. Hamilton, MA, MPH, Project Manager, Center on Mental Health Services Research & Policy, Department of Psychiatry, University of Illinois at Chicago, 104 South Michigan Avenue, Suite 900, Chicago, IL 60603 (E-mail: Mhamilton@psych.uic.edu).

The authors are grateful to Stan Sloan, Judith Perloff, the staff and clients of Chicago House, Dr. Bernard Turnock and Dr. Jesus Ramirez-Vallez for their contributions to this manuscript. The authors also would like to acknowledge Dr. Judith A. Cook and the UIC Center on Mental Health Services Research and Policy for support of this study.

This research was funded under the Field-Initiated Research Grant Program, No. H133G010093, United States Department of Education, National Institute on Disability & Rehabilitation Research.

The views expressed herein are those of the authors and do not necessarily reflect the policy or position of any Federal agency or the collaborating service organization.

[Haworth co-indexing entry note]: "The Relationship Between Type and Quality of Social Support and HIV Medication Adherence." Hamilton, Marie M., Lisa A. Razzano, and Nicole B. Martin. Co-published simultaneously in *the Journal of HIV/AIDS & Social Services* (The Haworth Press, Inc.) Vol. 6, No. 1/2, 2007, pp. 39-63; and: *HIV Treatment Adherence: Challenges for Social Services* (ed: Lana Sue Ka'opua and Nathan L. Linsk) The Haworth Press, Inc., 2007, pp. 39-63. Single or multiple copies of this article are available for a fee from The Haworth Document Delivery Service [1-800-HAWORTH, 9:00 a.m. - 5:00 p.m. (EST). E-mail address: docdelivery@haworthpress.com].

Available online at http://jhaso.haworthpress.com
doi: 10.1300/J187v06n01_04

factors affect adherence, including demographics, income, housing, mental health issues, and access to health care, as well as types and quality of social support. This paper summarizes results regarding specific sources of social support that are part of a larger, randomized study of medication adherence among people with HIV/AIDS. Results summarize findings from 98 program participants and include information regarding support from partners, family and health care providers, as well as the impact of support from these sources on medication adherence. Among participants in this study, those with higher levels of social support from partners demonstrated higher rates of medication adherence. Those who received more social support from their families, however, reported significantly lower adherence rates. These results suggest that efforts to improve medication adherence need to address the diverse types of social support networks of people diagnosed with HIV/AIDS. doi:10.1300/J187v06n01_04

[Article copies available for a fee from The Haworth Document Delivery Service: 1-800-HAWORTH. E-mail address: <docdelivery@haworthpress.com> Website: <http://www.HaworthPress.com> © 2007 by The Haworth Press, Inc. All rights reserved.]

KEYWORDS. HIV/AIDS, social support, adherence, health function

INTRODUCTION

Despite advances in HIV treatment, highly active antiretroviral therapy (HAART) continues to be characterized as one of the most complex pharmacological treatment strategies (Johnson et al., 2003; Nichols-English & Poirier, 2000). Individuals prescribed HAART take multiple tablets multiple times each day. Many regimens have other complex requirements: some must be stored under specific conditions; some must be taken with food or only on an empty stomach; and still others require that they be taken at times separate from other medications. In addition, many clients experience severe side effects from medications, such as lipodystrophy (i.e., a change in fat distribution, which can produce alterations in appearance including a protruding stomach, sunken eyes, and fat accumulation on the neck), chronic diarrhea, and fatigue that can also impact adherence (Chesney et al., 2000; Chesney, 2003). As a result, many continue to have difficulty managing these complicated medication regimens (Bangsberg et al., 2000). Currently, National

Institute of Health (NIH) guidelines indicate that optimal treatment benefit requires 95% adherence or higher from individuals taking HIV medications; less than 95% adherence is associated with the development of drug resistant strains of the virus that can eliminate treatment options for people living with HIV infection (Chesney, 2003; NIH, 2004; Patterson et al., 2000). Treatment resistant HIV not only is devastating to infected individuals, but also has deleterious effects on overall public health due to documented transmission of these multi-drug resistant strains through a population (Bogart, Catz, Kelly, & Benotsch, 2001; Miller & Hayes, 2000). Since antiretroviral medications require such a high degree of adherence, and the health risks associated with non-adherence are significant, improving adherence to HIV treatment regimens has become a critical issue to be addressed by HIV researchers, service providers and consumers.

Many factors have been shown to affect adherence, including regular and adequate income, stable housing, and health care (Miller & Hayes, 2000). Demographic characteristics themselves, such as race and gender also pose unique challenges with regard to adherence (Ferguson et al., 2002). Other reasons for poor adherence also have been cited, including: lack of social support (Gordillo, del Amo, Soriano, & González-Lahoz, 1999); health beliefs, such as high levels of health distress, fears related to unexpected health transitions, and limitations in social functioning related to chronic illness (Gao, Nau, Rosenbluth, Scott, & Woodward, 2000); lower education and poor health literacy (Kalichman, Ramachandran, & Catz, 1999); depression (Cook et al., 2004; Rabkin, Ferrando, Lin, Sewell, & McElhiney, 2000); other co-occurring mental illnesses (Kilbourne, Justice, Rabenck, Rodriguez-Barradas, & Weissman, 2001; Palmer, Salcedo, Miller, Winiarski, & Arno, 2003) and physical illnesses (Miller & Hayes, 2000); and substance abuse (Martini et al., 2004). While some of these factors are behavioral and potentially can be managed or controlled by the individual, others are the result of environmental factors or reflect more complex social dynamics. For example, support and assistance from family and friends may affect adherence as a result of reducing depression, providing practical assistance, promoting self-esteem and hope, and buffering the stresses associated with being ill (Shumaker & Hill, 1991). Therefore, in consideration of these factors, this paper examines relationships between different sources of social support and medication adherence among people living with HIV.

SOCIAL SUPPORT, HIV MEDICATION, AND TREATMENT ADHERENCE

Previous studies that have specifically examined the relationship between social support and HIV treatment adherence have found this relationship mediated by several factors. Overall, studies show that participants with lower rates of adherence report significantly lower levels of social support (Catz, Kelly, Bogart, Bonotsch, & McAuliffe, 2000; Gordillo et al., 1999). In other investigations, social support and treatment related self-efficacy contributed to long-term adherence and predicted nonadherence. Simoni, Frick, Lockhart, and Liebovitz et al. (2002) found that an identified need for social support was positively related to non-adherence. Based on their results, these authors suggest that both the need for support, as well as the lack of it, can interfere with achieving higher levels of adherence (Simoni et al.). The type of support provided, however, can take a variety of forms, such as relationships that are affirming, enhance and impart information, address spirituality, or provide empathic listening.

Source of social support also plays an important role in medication adherence. Studies have identified several viable sources of social support that may affect adherence, such as support from partners and healthcare providers. In one study, higher rates of medication adherence were associated with partner beliefs regarding lower perceived risk of HIV transmission, as well as associated with unprotected anal/vaginal sex within the couple (Wagner, Remien, Carballo-Dieguez, & Dolezal, 2002). Healthcare providers may also influence client's capacity to adhere to medication regimens. A qualitative study of individuals living with HIV (N = 28) who reported more positive relationships with primary care physicians tended to report higher levels of adherence, while more conflicted provider relationships tended to reduce adherence (Roberts, 2002).

The relationship between support from family members and medication adherence, however, is less clear. Overall, there are relatively few published quantitative investigations that specifically focus on issues related to family support relationships. One qualitative study of the relationship between HAART and disclosure of HIV status found that some individuals reported that family involvement promoted medication adherence (Klitzman et al., 2004). However, this article quoted only one individual, so it is difficult to know how many participants experienced this phenomenon. In addition, among other studies of family support in the literature, most focus on support provided to children living with HIV/AIDS from parents, rather than to adult family members. Support to adults living with HIV/AIDS from other family members is one of the focal issues in the present manuscript.

Finally, Gigliotti (2002) suggests that in addition to the source, certain types of social support are more effective in specific situations and more effective when specific people in the person's support network offer them. Gigliotti examines three functional types of social support using items from the Norbeck Social Support Questionnaire: "affect" (i.e., the expression of positive affect from one person towards another); "affirmation" (i.e., the endorsement of another person's behavior, beliefs, or expressed views); and "aid" (i.e., the giving of symbolic or tangible assistance). Gigliotti further suggests that by investigating specific sources and types of support, as well as unique characteristics of network distribution, researchers can gain a more comprehensive understanding of the role of overall social support.

STUDY PURPOSE

Thus, this paper explores the impact of three types of functional social support (i.e., affect, affirmation, and aid) on medication adherence. Data used in this analysis were generated from a larger, randomized intervention study examining the relationship between several factors related to medication adherence, including demographics, biological markers of illness progression, physical and mental health symptoms, and social support.

METHOD

Sampling and Participant Recruitment

The sample for this study consisted of 98 participants enrolled in the University of Illinois at Chicago (UIC) Medication Adherence Program Study (MAPS). Eligibility criteria for the MAPS included being 18 years of age or older, living with HIV infection or AIDS, currently taking medications for physical and/or mental health conditions, and ability to provide informed consent. In addition, all potential participants were required to be receiving services through Chicago House (a local AIDS service organization). Chicago House is a community organization that provides a variety of services to people living with HIV/AIDS, including case management, employment and job training, and housing. Some participants learned about the study through flyers posted at Chicago House, while other participants were informed of the study directly by case managers and other agency staff. Regardless of how participants learned about the MAPS, all were required to participate in a brief face-to-face recruitment meeting with the study coordinator in order to officially enroll and provide informed consent.

Based on services tracking data available from Chicago House, approximately 142 clients are active at the agency, but Chicago House does not specifically track use of medications for HIV or other health-related treatment. Thus, the eligible pool of participants was estimated to include all 142 active clients. However, based on a particular study eligibility criterion, only those Chicago House service clients taking medications were eligible to join the study. Over the course of the MAPS, a final total of 98 individuals participated in the study.

As noted in Table 1, 71% of participants were male (n = 70), 26% were women (n = 25), and 3% (n = 3) identified as male-to-female transgendered individuals. The racial/ethnic groups represented in the study were African American (48%, n = 47), Caucasian (37%, n = 36), Latino/Hispanic (7%, n = 7), and Hawaiian/Pacific Islander (2%, n = 2). Six percent (n = 6) identified as having a multi-racial identity or as members of other racial/ethnic groups. Twenty-five percent of the participants

TABLE 1. Participant Demographic Characteristics at Baseline (N = 98)*

Characteristics	n	%
Gender		
Male	70	71
Female	25	26
Transgender[a]	3	3
Race/Ethnicity		
African American	47	48
White/Caucasian	36	37
Latino/Hispanic	7	7
Asian/Pacific Islander	2	2
Other/Multi-Racial	6	6
Education		
Less than high school	25	25
High school graduate/GED	28	29
Some college or technical training	29	30
College Graduate/Prof. Degree	16	16
Has Children	41	42
Men**	19	27
Women**	22	79

Average Number *Co-Resident* Children** 1 (median = 0, range 0-7)
[a] All participants identified as transitioning from male-to-female.
* Variations in sample size are the result of missing data.
**Among those who reported having children only.

had not completed high school (n = 25), 29% (n = 28) were high school graduates, 30% (n = 29) completed some college or achieved technical or Associate's degrees, and 16% (n = 16) completed college or received professional degrees (e.g., Masters). Forty-two percent (n = 41) reported having children, with an average of one co-resident child. Detailed analyses of baseline interview data, including chi square, t-tests, and analysis of variance depending on the nature of the variables tested, showed no significant differences between participants randomized into the intervention and comparison groups on relevant study characteristics, including demographics, level of HIV medication adherence, impairment from symptoms of HIV/AIDS, use of alcohol and other drugs, or any of the other study outcomes.

Procedures

These data on social support and medication adherence were collected from participants at baseline and again six months later. Once participants were informed of the nature of their participation and provided written informed consent, they completed baseline interviews with trained MAPS project interviewers. Interviews were conducted during face-to-face meetings, in private settings away from case management staff, and were approximately 45 to 60 minutes in duration. For their participation in interviews, program participants were compensated with vouchers for use at a local grocery store or for transit authority fares for their participation in the interviews. Upon completion of the interview, participants were randomly assigned to either the MAPS intervention condition or the comparison condition (i.e., case management services-as-usual from Chicago House). The present analysis describes data related to social support findings and their relationship to medication adherence among MAPS study participants at baseline and six months later. Between baseline and six-months, a follow-up rate exceeding 95% was maintained over the course of the project.

Intervention

The UIC MAPS intervention included several components, including: two educational workshops addressing the use of antiretroviral medications, treatment planning, maintaining health, detecting early symptoms of illness progression, etc.; the development of individualized medication plans (I-MAPs) and individualized medication and treatment planning meetings with clients. Participants met with a medication specialist three times per month for a period of four months, for a total of 16 individualized contacts. This analysis does not, however, explore the impact of the adherence intervention program itself and its effects, if any, on study participants, except as they relate to its relationship to the type and quality of the social support these clients reported.

Instrumentation

The MAPS protocol collected detailed information regarding demographic characteristics, medication adherence, and social support. The instruments used to measure medication adherence and social support are described below.

Adult AIDS Clinical Trials Group (ACTG) Adherence Baseline & Follow Up Questionnaires. The Adult AIDS Clinical Trials Group (AACTG) Adherence Baseline & Follow Up Questionnaires (AACTG-B and AACTG-F, respectively) are comprised of items examining multiple aspects of medication and treatment adherence. Respondents provided general information about the total number of missed medication dosages as well as the last time medications were skipped (e.g., within past two days, past two weeks, 2-4 weeks ago, 1-3 months ago). In cases where they indicated that medications were skipped, respondents were asked to rate 14 different reasons (e.g., simply forgot, not at home) why they missed a medication using a four-point scale (never, rarely, sometimes, often). Both the baseline and follow up measures also include indicators of adherence self-efficacy, beliefs about medication effectiveness, social support, and alcohol and drug use. Several studies have demonstrated that the ACTG-B and ACTG-F identify significant predictors of non-adherence in HIV/AIDS as well as other chronic illnesses (Chesney et al., 2000; Wainberg & Freidland, 1998).

Norbeck Social Support Questionnaire. The Norbeck Social Support Questionnaire is a 20-item instrument that measures multiple dimensions of social support, including items related to three types of functional support: affect, affirmation, and aid. "Affect" is defined as the expression of positive affect from one person towards another; "affirmation" is the endorsement another person's behavior, beliefs, or expressed views; and "aid" involves the giving of symbolic or tangible assistance (Gigliotti, 2002). Both affect and affirmation can be categorized as emotional support measures (Gigliotti; Norbeck, 1995). In the questionnaire, participants are asked to identify sources of support from friends, family, work or school, and other social networks. Each type of functional support is assessed by two questions. Participants are asked to rate each identified individual on a scale from 1 (not at all) to 5 (a great deal) with regard to how much support they provide for each of the three types of functional support. The measure has stable reliability and validity coefficients and has been used in published studies exploring the relationship between social support and health issues. Internal consistency for the current sample exceeded .80.

Outcome and Independent Variables

All relevant demographic information (e.g., gender, race/ethnicity), potential mode of transmission, and other characteristics were documented. Focal study outcome variables included indicators related to types and nature of social support (measured by the Norbeck Social Support Scale) and adherence (measured with the ACTG questionnaires). Since this analysis focused on support provided specifically by a partner, family members, and healthcare providers, the impact of any social support provided by friends is examined in another paper currently in preparation.

Although, many previous studies have suggested that support provided by friends and peers is more helpful than other types of support, these findings may result from an individual's ability to choose to pursue friendships that are more satisfying and rewarding. However, family support may have more influence on particular health domains. For example, Serovich, Kimberly, Mosack, and Lewis (2001) report that although women indicated that friends were more supportive overall, family support was more indicative of positive mental health and other factors. In addition, lower levels of family support have been linked to increased HIV risk taking for men who have sex with men ([MSMs]; Heckman, Kelly, & Somlai, 1998). Based on these issues, as well as an interest in examining less studied factors in the social support literature, the present analysis focuses on the relationship between medication adherence and social support from family (including partners) and health care providers.

Adherence was characterized in several ways. First, this outcome was defined by creating a dichotomous indicator that grouped all clients who reported 100% adherence versus those reporting 99% or less (i.e., 100% adherence = 1 vs. adherence < 100% = 0). Since drug resistance is associated with less than 95% adherence, anything less than perfect adherence was categorized as nonadherence for the purposes of this evaluation based on current NIH guidelines (NIH, 2004). In addition, adherence also was characterized using the number of reasons for not taking their medication as prescribed cited by participants in response to the ACTG questionnaire. The number of potential reasons on the ACTG ranged from 0 (none) to 14 (all of those listed). In addition to individual reasons cited for nonadherence overall, the frequency at which doses were missed as a result of specific reasons also was measured using a Likert-type scale ranging from 0 (never) to 4 (often). Gender also was dichotomized for use in analyses. In this case transgendered participants were included in these analyses as female participants, since this was how they identified their gender. The small number of transgendered individuals in the study did not impact the significance of the findings, since confirmatory analysis excluding these individuals were also conducted. Similarly, dichotomous variables were constructed for race/ethnicity, such that one pair divided all minorities (1) vs. whites (0), while the second paired African-Americans (1) vs. all other groups (0), since African-Americans comprised the largest proportion of people in the study.

Social support indicators also were characterized in several ways. The variable "*any* social support" was constructed by identifying participants who reported receiving support from any identified source. This strategy simply categorized individuals who received no support from an identified source as (0) along with those who reported receiving support (1). "Proportion of social support" was calculated by analyzing whether participants received "any support" from a specific source compared to how much support they received from all identified sources. Using proportions, instead of averages or mean values, allows responses to be evaluated using the same type of quantification, i.e., proportions are based on each participant's individual types of support (in the numerator) and their total from *all sources* of support (in the denominator). For example, one respondent with two family members out of four total sources (i.e., 2/4) as their pattern of support would have 50% from family; likewise, a participant with five family sources out of 10 (i.e., 5/10) also is characterized as 50%. In this example, if actual numbers for sources of support were used, the average (i.e., [2 + 5]/2 = 3.5) would not be the most representative value to describe the amount of support from family members. This coding strategy also was used to better characterize support received from any individual source. This is particularly relevant in the case of partner support, since unlike family or health care providers partners could be only one source within the total sources identified (e.g., 10% maximum, 1/10). Family or health care providers could have potentially been as much as 100% (i.e., 10/10) of sources identified among those with no spouse/partner.

Furthermore, as indicated by Gigliotti (2002), functional social support was calculated for each individual source of support by aggregating item ratings on specific Norbeck items in three areas: affect, affirmation, and aid. In this case, each new functional support values range from 0 (no support/low quality) to 5 (has support/high quality) reflecting more support as well as more positive ratings of the quality of that support. First ratings for each individual source were aggregated to produce a total score for that source. Next, these total scores among all sources of support listed were combined to reflect the total amount of support for each area. For example, to calculate a total family affect rating for an individual who listed three family sources of social support, ratings for each family source were calculated to produce an affect score. Next, all three affect scores were combined from all three sources to produce a total score for family affect.

Data Analyses

Data analyses included calculation of frequency distributions as well as descriptive and inferential statistics. In cases where distributions were not normal, statistical techniques (e.g., standard scores, conversion to square roots, use of logarithms) were applied to transform skewed distributions. For example, in skewed distributions, a higher proportion of scores are aggregated toward one end of the scale and taper off toward the other (Gravetter & Wallnau, 1992). As a result, skewed distributions can violate the statistical assumption of normal distribution, particularly among smaller samples.

Data aggregation was completed for nominal and ordinal variables where indicated, as well as to construct scales and total scores as instructed for the Norbeck and the ACTG adherence measures using procedures described in other published papers (Chesney et al., 2000; Gigliotti, 2002; Norbeck, Lindsey, & Carrieri, 1981). All analyses were designed to comply with guidelines from published papers that specify minimum requirements for statistical power, such as the number of cases per test variable (Kerlinger & Pedhauzer, 1973). All differences reported significant at $p < .05$ are summarized in the Results section. Calculations for percentages, cross-tabulations, and χ^2 analyses were conducted on the nominal and ordinal outcome variables of interest. Analysis of variance (ANOVA) was conducted with relevant study outcomes in order to identify any significant differences among continuous variables in the study. To detect changes over time among individual outcomes within- and between-groups, repeated-measures ANOVA (RM-ANOVA) was used. In addition, analyses considered unequal sample sizes between groups. In order to further reduce the probability of Type I errors that may result from multiple comparisons or non-normal distributions, appropriate adjustment procedures were conducted as described by Gravetter and Wallnau (1992), including use of Bonferroni procedures and adjustment (where indicated) of significance levels of the multiple ANOVAs conducted with these data. Appropriate correlations were used to determine relevant relationships among these types of factors.

RESULTS

Adherence to HIV Treatment

Results regarding reported adherence at the two time points are summarized in Table 2. As listed in the table, at baseline, 25% (n = 24) of study participants reported that they did not miss any medications (i.e., 100% adherence), while 75% (n = 74) missed at least one or more doses. On average, the number of individual reasons cited by participants for missing medication at baseline was 4, with a median also equal to 4. The average overall frequency of missed doses in the past 30 days at baseline was 7, with a median of 6, ranging from 0 (no reasons cited for missed doses) to 25 (several reasons cited with high frequency of missing doses). At the six-month interview, the number of participants reporting nonadherence in the past 30 days increased to 83% (n = 81), while the average number of reasons cited for missing medication decreased slightly to 3, with a median of 2. The range of missed doses

TABLE 2. Participants' Reported Reasons & Frequency of Missed Doses

Indicators of Nonadherence (N = 98)	Baseline		6-month	
	n	%	n	%
Any Missed Medications in Past 30 Days	74	75	81	83
Average Number of Reasons per person (median)	4(4)		3(2)	
Min/Max	(0-14)		(0-14)	
Overall Average Frequency of Missed Dosages (median)	7(6)		6(4)	
Min/Max	(0-25)		(0-29)	

remained the same, 0 to 14. The overall frequency of missed doses also decreased slightly to a mean of 6 (median = 4) missed dosages, while the range for the frequency of missed doses was 0 to 29.

Social Support

Frequencies and other descriptive information regarding outcomes related to social support are summarized in Table 3. Overall, the 98 participants identified three important sources of social support: spouses/partners, families and health care providers. At baseline, 19% (n = 18) of MAPS participants reported any social support from a spouse/partner, which, on average, represented 5% of their total sources of support. These findings were stable over time; 20% (n = 19) of participants reported support from a spouse/partner at T2. However, families were the source of support identified most frequently by all study participants. Almost half of study participants reported any support from family at baseline (47%, n = 46), and family support accounted for 36% of the total social support available to participants. At T2, approximately

TABLE 3. Summary of Sources and Types of Participant's Social Support

Kind of Social Support	Baseline		6-month	
	n	%	n	%
Spouse/Partner–Any Support Reported	**18**	**19**	**19**	**20**
Proportion of Total Support	5	5	5	5
Men	4	4	7	7
Women	7	7	7	2
Minorities	6	6	4	4
Non-Minorities	4	4	8	8
Family–Any Support Reported	**46**	**47**	**65**	**66**
Percentage of Total Support	**35**	**36**	**36**	**37**
Men	27	28	28	29
Women	39	40	57	58
Minorities	38	39	42	43
Non-Minorities	30	31	25	25
Health Care Provider–Any Support Reported	**39**	**40**	**37**	**38**
Percentage of Total Support	18	18	12	12
Men	17	17	13	13
Women	18	18	11	11
Minorities	19	19	10	10
Non-Minorities	15	15	17	17

two-thirds of respondents (66%, n = 65) reported family support. It is interesting to note, however, that although more participants were receiving support from their family at T2, family support comprised a smaller percentage of total overall support reported, at, on average, 31%. A sizeable number of participants also reported receiving support from health care providers. At baseline, 40% (n = 39) of respondents stated they received support from a doctor, nurse, case manager, or psychologist. Support from this source accounted for 18% of total social support. At T2, 38% (n = 37) of participants reported receiving support from a health care provider, and this support constituted 20% of the overall support reported.

Descriptive statistics characterizing ratings for "quality" of the three types of functional support (i.e., affect, affirmation, and aid) measured using the Norbeck are summarized in Table 4. Using the scoring method outlined by Gigliotti (2002), these values were computed for all participants regardless of whether they listed particular sources, since not having a specific source is a relevant and potentially important finding. Regarding functional support from partners, participants reported an average of 1.8 as the average rating for each of these types of functional support. In fact, median value was 0 since the majority of participants did not list a partner. These findings appear stable over time. At 6 months the average ratings for the different types of support remain similar:

TABLE 4. Summary of Ratings of Functional Support by Source[a]

Kind of Social Support	Baseline		6-month	
	Mean	Min/Max	Mean	Min/Max
Type of Partner/Spousal Support				
Affect	1.8	1-10	1.9	1-10
Affirmation	1.8	1-10	1.7	1-10
Aid	1.8	1-10	1.9	1-10
Type of Family Support				
Affect	12.7	1-83	15.3	1-100
Affirmation	11.4	1-90	13.9	1-99
Aid	10.4	1-64	12.5	1-90
Type of Health Care Provider Support				
Affect	5.2	1-59	5.1	1-50
Affirmation	5.0	1-57	4.7	1-43
Aid	4.3	1-50	4.0	1-30

[a] Higher functional support values reflect more positive support ratings.

affect (1.9), affirmation (1.7), and aid (1.9). With regard to functional support provided from families, the average values reported for each kind of support were similar to one another at baseline: affect (12.7), affirmation, (11.8), and aid (10.4). However, there were slight increases in these average ratings for family functional support over time (at 6-month): affect (15.3), affirmation (13.9), and aid (12.5). Health care providers also were a viable source of functional support. Average ratings for types of support from health care providers were: affect (5.2), affirmation (5.0), and aid (4.3). The ratings regarding the type of support provided at T2 were similar: affect (5.1), affirmation (4.7), and aid (4.0).

Zero-Order Relationships Among Social Support and Medication Adherence

Pearson correlations were conducted to determine the relationship between sources and kinds of social support and the adherence indicators. A zero-order correlation describes the predictive relationship between two variables only, ignoring the influence of other factors. Initial comparisons revealed a significant, negative relationship between spousal support and medication adherence. At baseline, as the proportion of partner support increased, the number of reasons for nonadherence, as well as the overall frequency of missed dosages decreased [$r(63) = -.31$, $p < .01$ and $r(62) = -.32$, $p < .01$, respectively]. These relationships persisted six months later; reasons for nonadherence were significantly fewer for participants receiving more support from a partner, $r(83) = -.23$, $p < .04$, and overall frequency of missed dosages was lower as well, $r(83) = -.25$, $p < .03$.

Although spousal/partner support had a positive impact on medication adherence, analyses of family support revealed that this source of support had a *negative* effect on medication adherence. Despite no initial relationships between each adherence indicator and family support at baseline, at T2 a significant, positive correlational relationship was identified. In particular, as the proportion of family support increased, the number of reasons for nonadherence also increased [$r(83) = .24$, $p < .03$], as did the frequency of missed doses [$r(79) = .23$, $p < .04$]. Support from health care providers initially demonstrated a significant positive relationship to nonadherence, however this relationship changed over time. At baseline, as the proportion of support from a healthcare provider increased, frequency of missed dosages also increased, $r(62) = .28$, $p < .03$. At T2, however, this relationship was no longer significant. Furthermore, there were no relationships between the number of reasons cited for missed doses and the proportion of support from a health care provider at either baseline or T2.

Next, relationships between the source of support and each type of functional support were examined. With regard to spousal/partner support overall, significant relationships were identified for each of the individual functional areas and number of reasons cited for non-adherence: affect [$r(98) = -.27, p < .01$]; affirmation [$r(98) = .26, p < .01$]; and aid [$r(98) = -.26, p < .01$]. At T2, however, no relationship between functional support from a partner and reasons for nonadherence was identified. The type of functional support received from a partner/spouse at T1 also was significantly related to overall frequency of *missed dosages*: affect, $r(80) = -.28, p < .01$; affirmation, $r(80) = -.27, p < .02$; and aid, $r(80) = -.29, p < .01$. At T2, partner support continued to have positive effects on missed dosages, such that higher levels of partner functional support were related to lower frequency of reported missed doses: affect [$r(95) = -.28, p < .01$], affirmation [$r(95) = -.27, p < .01$], and aid [$r(95) = -.27, p < .01$].

The quality and type of functional support provided by the *family*, were not related to adherence at baseline; at T2, however, a significant positive relationship was present between the kind and quality of family functional support and nonadherence. The number of reasons for missing medication doses was related to affect [$r(98) = .46, p < .01$], affirmation [$r(98) = .48, p < .01$] and aid [$r(98) = .45, p < .01$], as well as the overall frequency of missed doses: affect [$r(80) = .34, p < .01$]; affirmation [$r(80) = .35, p < .01$]; and aid [$r(80) = .33, p < .01$]. Thus, as the quality and kind of social support from family increased, nonadherence to medication regimens measured with two independent indictors also increased, revealing a potentially negative effect of family support on adherence.

Finally, functional support from a healthcare provider was also related to both adherence indicators at baseline. The total number of reasons for missed dosages was positively related to functional support from a healthcare provider: affect [$r(98) = .29, p < .01$], affirmation [$r(98) = .27, p < .01$], and aid [$r(98) = .28, p < .01$]. In addition, significant correlations were found between overall frequency of missed dosages and type of functional support provided by health care providers; affect [$r(95) = .27, p < .01$], affirmation [$r(95) = .25, p < .05$], and aid [$r(95) = .25, p < .05$]. At T2, however, there were no significant relationships between these factors.

In order to examine racial and ethnic differences in sources of and quality of social support, one-way repeated measures analysis of variance

(RM-ANOVA) was utilized. In the first analysis comparing minorities to non-minority whites on average proportion of support provided, no main effect for race was demonstrated for partner or health care provider support. There were multiple effects, however, revealed for family support. A within-subjects main effect for race/ethnicity was revealed by time, such that between the time of study entry and six months later, non-minority whites reported that a significantly lower proportion of their support was from family members compared to minority participants (25% vs. 43%), $F(1, 82) = 7.3, p < .01$.

These multivariate tests also revealed effects for the three different types of functional support. First, minorities received more positive *affect* support overall, $F(1, 96) = 10.2, p < .01$. Over time, within-subjects effects also indicated that positive affect support from family *decreased* among whites, but *increased* among minorities, $F(1, 96) = 5.5, p < .02$. Findings regarding *affirmation* functional support were similar; overall, minorities had more family affirmation than non-minority whites ($F(1, 96) = 9.8, p < .01$) and over time, family affirmation among whites decreased while minority family affirmation increased $F(1, 96) = 5.5$, $p < .02$. *Aid* functional support from family also followed this pattern; functional aid from families was significantly greater for minority participants than for non-minority whites overall, $F(1, 96) = 12.1, p < .001$, while aid support from family decreased over time for whites but increased among minorities, $F(1, 96) = 4.5, p < .04$.

Analyses were also conducted to determine the effects of gender on the social support indicators. A within-subjects effect for gender was detected for partner/spousal support (i.e., an effect by time). In particular, women received a significantly larger proportion of their support from a partner/spouse at baseline than at T2 (6% vs. 2%), $F(1, 50) = p < .03$; men, in contrast, received a lower proportion of support from a partner/spouse at baseline, but that proportion increased over time (4% vs. 7%). Furthermore, a within-subjects effect also was revealed for family support such that both men and women received a higher proportion of their overall support from their families at T2 than other potential sources, $F(1,50) = 6.4, p < .01$. However, in this case, women experienced a greater increase in the total proportion of support provided by their families than men (58% vs. 29%), $F(1,50) = 4.5, p < .04$. There was no effect found for overall or functional support from healthcare providers by gender.

Significant effects were reported for all three measures of functional support by gender. First, men received significantly more functional support from a partner over time: affect ($F(1, 96) = 7.3, p < .01$); affirmation

(F(1, 96) = 7.3, $p < .01$); and aid (F(1, 96) = 6.8, $p < .03$). Thus, women had significantly less overall spousal support, and they also reported being less likely to maintain partner support over time. There was also a main effect demonstrated for gender and family support; however, women received a larger proportion of their functional support from their families than men, F(1,50) = 6.9, $p < .01$. Like other findings in this paper, family support on all three functional support variables fluctuated over time: affect, F(1, 96) = 5.4, $p < .02$; affirmation, F(1, 96) = 5.7, $p < .02$; and aid, F(1, 96) = 6.9, $p < .04$. In each case, women received significantly more affect, affirmation, and aid support from their families than men six months after joining the study. As noted for other analyses, no significant effects were revealed for support from healthcare providers.

DISCUSSION

The relationship between antiretroviral medication adherence and social support is complex. Different sources of support dramatically impact participants' rates of adherence. Overall, partner support was associated with increased adherence, both in reducing the number of doses missed and the number of reasons cited for missing doses. In addition, this support was stable over time, and better functional support seemed to lead to better adherence. Unfortunately, only 20% of MAPS participants had access to this type of support. The role of partner support did not seem to differ across ethnicity or racial backgrounds. However, partner support also was affected by participant's gender, such that women experienced significantly lower partner support over time compared to men. The information collected in this study, however, does not allow for a comprehensive examination of the complex issues related to partner support. Although ratings of partner support from participants in this study were positively associated with adherence, it is essential that future studies examine partner support with more detail in order to develop a better understanding of the specific characteristics of partner support and the exact nature of their relationship to medication adherence. Furthermore, some of these factors could be related to sexual orientation and the unique aspects of same-sex compared to heterosexual relationships. This project focused primarily on risk factors associated with mode of HIV infection rather than on sexual orientation per se, since individuals' behaviors may differ from the way they characterize their sexual activities. For example, many men identify as heterosexual despite the fact that they still engage in sex with other men. Clearly, future studies should examine more definitive information regarding heterosexual and same-sex partnerships in order to explore the complexity of the relationship between types of partners, partner support, and adherence.

Family support was the most commonly identified source of support by participants. This type of support was significantly higher among minority participants than non-minority whites, and this relationship became stronger over time. This finding supports earlier research that demonstrated that parents in African-American families have an increased capacity and readiness to care for disabled children in comparison to white parents (Pickett, Vraniak, Cook, & Cohler, 1993). This analysis also found that women received a higher proportion of their support from their families, and higher amount of functional support from their families than men. This also is congruent with previous research demonstrating that women's support systems are more oriented toward family ties than men's (Pinto & McKay, 2004).

Surprisingly, however, higher levels of support from family were associated with increased number of doses missed and more reasons cited for missing doses. It is unlikely that this relationship is a result of conflicted family relationships since participants rated the quality of the functional support they received as very positive. However, it is possible that extended family networks can cause increased strain due to demands on time and energy (Pickett et al., 1993), which subsequently could impact adherence. This positive association between family support and medication non-adherence is particularly troubling, as participants received a higher percentage of their overall support from family members over time. Thus, as this proportion of family support increased, adherence decreased. The consequences of this relationship also may disproportionally affect minority participants and women, since both groups reported receiving a larger proportion of their total social support from their families.

Another factor that may account for this problematic association is non-disclosure of HIV status. If a person's family is not aware that a member is living with HIV, the family cannot provide support related to medication adherence, and the effort exerted to keep this information secret can negatively impact adherence. Hiding one's HIV status can lead to missed doses and reduced adherence, since taking HAART medications may 'out' infected individuals (Klitzman et al., 2004). Although study participants highly rated their satisfaction level with support from families, it is plausible that this satisfaction level did not result in disclosure of HIV status. Serovich, Ebensen, and Mason (2005) found that as satisfaction with a family relationship decreases, the rate of disclosure increased. Therefore, some individuals may not disclose their status because they do not want to risk losing the family support that they currently receive. Furthermore, disclosure to children may be particularly hard for women, even though it appears that non-disclosure may impact adherence. Mellins, Kang, Leu, Havens, and Chesney (2003) found that less disclosure to children regarding HIV status was associated with reduced adherence to follow-up medical appointments for women living with HIV. Women may not want to burden their children with fears and concerns that are likely to result from disclosure of their HIV status (Sowell, Seals, Phillips, & Julious, 2003). Also, younger children could inadvertently disclose a parent's HIV status without understanding the ramifications of such a disclosure (Sandowski, Lambe, & Barroso, 2004); this may be another reason parents may not have discussed their health with their children. Anecdotally, research interviewers for this study reported that many children seemed to be uninformed of their parent's HIV status since research interviews were interrupted and paused when children entered the room. Many parents in the study lived with their children, so this could make it even more challenging to maintain secrecy around one's HIV status. Unfortunately, the MAPS study did not measure disclosure within families among participants because this potential relationship had not been identified when the study was initially designed. Failure to measure disclosure is a limitation of this study, and future investigations should specifically address disclosure and level of support from family members.

Although, many studies have focused on the importance of the impact of relationships with health care providers on medication adherence (Chesney et al., 2000; Stone et al., 1998), this impact is not as strongly demonstrated by results from this study. Participants who identified receiving a higher proportion of their social support from healthcare providers were significantly more likely to *miss* dosages than other individuals. However, over time this relationship disappeared. This may result from extra support that health care providers may give to individuals who have demonstrated more noteworthy problems with treatment adherence. If patients have experienced difficulty following previously prescribed treatment regimens, health care providers may be more involved in that individual's care in an effort to address adherence issues. It is heartening to see, as well, that over time the increased support from providers no longer results in higher rates of nonadherence. Thus, it appears over time although there is no longer a significant relationship between health care provider social support and missed dosages, the relationship has moved in a more positive direction.

Findings from this study also suggest that despite specific types of functional support including affect, affirmation, and aid, the source of any of these three types of support appears to be most relevant to medication adherence. Although differences between partners, families, and healthcare providers as sources of support were revealed as part of this evaluation, participants who received one form of functional support were also likely to report support in the other functional areas. Most importantly, however, these findings also suggest that sources of functional support may be different based on demographic factors, such as race/ethnicity and gender. Among minorities and women, families are the predominant source of functional support. However, men were more likely to report partners as a source of functional support.

Overall findings from this analysis suggest the need for more research on the relationship between sources and types of social support, adherence and other mediating factors, such as demographics. In particular, it would be important for future studies to examine the potentially mediating role of disclosure on social support and medication adherence. Identifying whether social support sources are aware of an individual's HIV status would greatly assist in better understanding the impact of disclosure on social support. In addition, since adherence has been described as a dynamic process that changes over time in relation to the lives, attitudes, emotions and beliefs of the individuals living with HIV (Remien et al., 2003), it would be important to further explore the role of social support and medication adherence over a longer time frame, such as one year or longer. This would help to better understand how the relationship between medication adherence and social support changes over time.

There are several strengths and limitations in this study that also should be noted. One strength of the study is the gender composition of the participants. In contrast to other investigations in the field, this evaluation includes a higher proportion of women participants. Thus, these findings can be generalized beyond reports that have included primarily men or with subsamples of women too small to support inferential analysis. In addition, few studies have specifically examined the source and kind of social support and its relationship to HIV medication adherence. This evaluation raises important questions regarding the negative impact that some sources of social support can have on medication adherence. However, the study was not able to examine differences based on gender and ethnicity simultaneously. Clearly, future studies should more closely examine these issues with larger samples, those with larger groups of women overall, and those with more ethnically diverse groups of women. In addition, this analysis focused on support provided by a partner, family members, and healthcare providers, but did not examine the impact of any social support provided by friends. Future studies should examine the role of peer support overall, as well as the influence of functional peer support in the areas of affect, affirmation and aid on adherence. It may be especially important to do so in order to determine whether peer support varies overall, as well as with respect to gender and among different racial/ethnic groups.

CONCLUSION

The findings of this study suggest that efforts to improve medication adherence need to include the social support networks of people diagnosed with HIV/AIDS. Adherence interventions need to work with identified sources of support to increase their knowledge regarding the importance of HIV treatment adherence and the potentially severe health outcomes that can result from nonadherence. In addition, it seems important to provide specific strategies that sources of support can utilize to promote better adherence in their loved ones. These interventions may also need to address concerns regarding disclosure for those living with HIV, and assist individuals living with HIV to identify potentially supportive members of their social network. In the event that individuals are not able to disclose to people in their support network, interventions should help address how to manage the illness and treatment while maintaining this secret.

It seems equally important to reduce the stigma associated with HIV. Individuals living with HIV are afraid to disclose their status because they fear rejection. Interventions must continue to educate the public about HIV and work to create greater empathy and support within communities. Providing education and stigma reduction programs to churches and social organizations in communities of color seems particularly important given the results regarding the higher rates of support provided by family members found in this study. This type of programming may help individuals to feel more comfortable disclosing their status and may assist families in providing support more specifically related to HIV and medication adherence issues.

REFERENCES

Bangsberg, D. R., Hecht, F. M., Charlebois, E. D., Zolopa, A. R., Holodniy, M., Sheiner, L. et al. (2000). Adherence to protease inhibitors, HIV-1 viral load, and development of drug resistance in an indigent population. *AIDS, 14*, 357-366.

Bogart, L. M., Catz, S. L., Kelly, J. A., & Benotsch, E. G. (2001). Factors influencing physicians' judgments of adherence and treatment decisions for patients with HIV disease. *Medical Decision Making,* 21(1), 28-36

Catz, S. L, Kelly, J. A., Bogart, L. M., Benotsch, E. G., & McAuliffe, T. L. (2000). Patterns, correlates, and barriers to medication adherence among persons prescribed new treatments from HIV disease. *Health Psychology,* 19(2), 124-133.

Chesney, M. (2003). Review: Adherence to HAART regimens. *AIDS Patient Care and STDs,* 17(4), 169-177.

Chesney, M. A., Ickovics, J. R., Chambers, D. B., Gifford, A. L., Neidig, J., Zwickl, B. et al. (2000). Self-reported adherence to antiretroviral medications among participants in HIV clinical trials: The AACTG Adherence Instruments. *AIDS Care,* 12(3), 255-266.

Cook, J. A., Grey, D. D., Burke, J. K. Cohen, M. H., Gurtman, A. C., Richardson, J. L. et al. (2004). Depressive symptoms and AIDS-related mortality among a multisite cohort of HIV-positive women. *American Journal of Public Health,* 94(7), 1133-1140.

Ferguson, T. F., Stewart, K. E., Funkhouser, E., Tolson, J., Westfall, A. O., & Saag, M. S. (2002). Patient-perceived barriers to antiretroviral adherence: Associations with race. *AIDS Care,* 14(5), 607-617.

Gao, X., Nau, D. P., Rosenbluth, S. A., Scott, V., Woodward, C. (2000). The relationship of disease severity, health beliefs and medication adherence among HIV patients. *AIDS Care, 12,* 387-398.

Gigliotti, E. (2002). A confirmation of the factor structure of the Norbeck Social Support Questionnaire. *Nursing Research, 51*(5), 276-284.

Gordillo, V., del Amo, J., Soriano, V., & González-Lahoz, J. (1999). Sociodemographic and psychological variables influencing adherence to antiretroviral therapy. *AIDS,* 13(13), 1763-1769.

Gravetter, F. J., & Wallnau, L. B. (1992). *Statistics for the behavioral sciences, third edition.* St. Paul, MN: West Publishing Company.

Heckman, T. G., Kelly, J. A., & Somlai, A. M. (1998). Predictors of continued high-risk behavior in a community sample of persons living with HIV/AIDS. *AIDS and Behavior,* 2(2), 127-135.

Johnson, M. O., Catz, S. L., Remein, R. H., Rotheram-Borus, M. J., Morin, S. F., Charlebois, E. et al. (2003). Theory-guided, empirically supported avenues for intervention on HIV medication nonadherence: Findings from the Health Living Project. *AIDS Patient Care and STDs,* 17(12), 645-656.

Kalichman, S. C., Ramachandran, B., & Catz, S. (1999). Adherence to combination antiretroviral therapies in HIV patients of low health literacy. *Journal of General Internal Medicine, 14*(5), 267-273.

Kerlinger, F., & Pedhazur, F. N., (1973). *Multiple regression in behavioral research.* New York, NY: Holt, Rinehart, & Winston.

Kilbourne, A. M., Justice, A. C., Rabeneck, L., Rodriguez-Barradas, M., & Weissman, S. (2001). General medical and psychiatric co-morbidity among HIV-infected veterans in the post-HAART era. *Journal of Clinical Epidemiology, 54,* S22-S28.

Klitzman, R. L., Kirshembaum, S. B., Dodge, B., Remien, R. H., Ehrhardt, A. A., Johnson, M. O. et al. (2004). Intricacies and inter-relationships between HIV disclosure and HAART: A qualitative study. *AIDS Care, 16*(5), 628-640.

Martini, M., Recchia, E., Nasta, P., Castanotto, D., Chiaffarino, F., Parazzini, F. et al. (2004). Illicit drug use: Can it predict adherence to antiretroviral therapy? *European Journal of Epidemiology, 19*, 585-587.

Mellins, C. A., Kang, E., Leu, C. S., Havens, J. L., & Chesney, M. A. (2003). Longitudinal study of mental health and psychosocial predictors of medical treatment adherence in mothers living with HIV disease. *AIDS Patient Care and STDs, 17*(8), 407-416.

Miller, L. G., & Hayes, R. D. (2000). Adherence to combination antiretroviral therapy: Synthesis of literature and clinical implications. *The AIDS Reader, 10*(3), 177-185.

National Institutes of Health. (2004). Guidelines for the use of antiretroviral agents in HIV-1 infected adults and adolescents. Retrieved December 1, 2005 from http://aidsinfo.nih.gov/ContentFiles/AdultandAdolescentGL_AdherenceSup.pdf

Nichols-English, G., & Poirier, S. (2000). Optimizing adherence to pharmaceutical care plans. *Journal of the American Pharmaceutical Association, 40*(4), 475-85.

Norbeck, J. S. (1995). Who is our consumer? Shaping nursing programs to meet emerging needs. *Journal of Professional Nursing, 11*(6), 325-31.

Norbeck, J. S., Lindsey, A. M., & Carrieri, V. L. (1981). The development of an instrument to measure social support. *Nursing Research, 30*(5), 264-269.

Palmer, N. B., Salcedo, J, Miller, A. L., Winiarski, M., & Arno, P. (2003). Psychiatric and social barriers to HIV medication adherence in a triply diagnosed methadone population. *AIDS Patient Care and STDs, 17*(12), 635-644.

Paterson, D. L., Swindells, S., Mohr J., Brester, M., Vergis, E. N., Squier, C. et al. (2000). Adherence to protease inhibitor therapy and outcomes in patients with HIV infection. *Annals of Internal Medicine, 133*, 21-30.

Pickett, S. A., Vraniak, D. A., Cook, J. A., & Cohler, B. J. (1993). Strength in adversity: Blacks bear burden better than whites. *Professional Psychology: Research and Practice, 24*(4), 460-467.

Pinto, R. M., & McKay, M. M. (2004). Do age and gender of social supports matter for low-income African-American women attending an HIV prevention program? *Journal of HIV/AIDS & Social Services, 3*(2), 5-25.

Rabkin, J. G., Ferrando, S. J., Lin, S., Sewell, M., & McElhiney, M. (2000). Psychological effects of HAART: A 2-year study. *Psychosomatic Medicine, 62*(3), 413-422.

Remien, R. H., Hirky, A. E., Johnson, M. O., Weinhardt, L. S., Whittier, D., & Le, G. M. (2003). Adherence to medication treatment: A qualitative study of facilitators and barriers among a diverse sample of HIV + men and women in four cities. *AIDS and Behavior, 7*(1), 61-72.

Roberts, K. J. (2002). Physician-patient relationships, patient satisfaction, and antiretroviral medication adherence among HIV-infected adults attending a public health clinic. *AIDS Patient Care and STDs, 16*(1), 43-50.

Sandowski, M., Lambe, C., & Barroso, J. (2004). Stigma in HIV-positive women. *Journal of Nursing Scholarship, 36*(2), 122-8.

Serovich, J. M., Ebensen, A. J., & Mason, T. L. (2005). HIV disclosure by men who have sex with men to immediate family over time. *AIDS Patient Care and STDs, 19*(8), 506-517.

Serovich, J. M., Kimberly, J. A., Mosack, K. E., & Lewis, T. L. (2001). The role of family and friend social support in reducing emotional distress among HIV-positive women. *AIDS Care, 13*(3), 335-341.

Shumaker, S. A., & Hill, D. R. (1991). Gender differences in social support and physical health. *Health Psychology,10,* 102-111.

Simoni, J. M, Frick, P. A., Lockhart, D., & Liebovitz, D. (2002). Mediators of social support and antiretroviral adherence among an indigent population in New York City. *AIDS Patient Care and STDs, 16*(9), 431-439.

Sowell, R. L., Seals, B. F, Phillips, K. D., & Julious, C. H. (2003). Disclosure of HIV infection: How do women decide to tell? *Health Education Research, 18*(1), 32-44.

Stone, V. E., Clarke, J., Lovell, J., Steger, K. A., Hirschhorn, L. R., Boswell, S. et al. (1998). HIV/AIDS patients' perspectives on adhering to regimens containing protease inhibitors. *Journal of General Internal Medicine, 13,* 586-93.

Wagner, G. J., Remien, R. H., Carballo-Dieguez, A., & Dolezal, C. (2002). Correlates of adherence to combination antiretroviral therapy among members of HIV-positive mixed status couples. *AIDS Care, 14*(1), 105-109.

Wainberg, M. A., & Freidland, G. (1998). Public health implications of antiretroviral therapy and HIV drug resistance. *Journal of the American Medical Association, 279,* 1977-1983.

doi:10.1300/J187v06n01_04

Predictors of Medication Adherence Among HIV/AIDS Clients

Elizabeth C. Pomeroy, PhD, LCSW
Sanna Thompson, PhD, MSW
Kelly Gober, MSW
LaTonya Noel, MSW

SUMMARY. Lack of adherence to medication regimens among people living with HIV/AIDS can lead to new drug resistant strains of the virus as well as continuing spread of the disease. Due to suboptimal adherence, the prevalence of these resistant strains continues to increase, posing a serious public health risk. Adherence to the various medications must be 95-100% complete in order to be considered adequate; however, 57% to 77% of patients fail to reach this level of adherence. Treatment of HIV-infected persons with highly active antiretroviral therapy (HAART) is often challenging due to the presence of factors that can affect adherence, such as complex regimens, total pill burden, and food dosing restrictions.

Elizabeth C. Pomeroy, PhD, LCSW, is a Professor; Sanna Thompson, PhD, MSW, is an Associate Professor in the Substance Abuse Research Development Program; and Kelly Gober, MSW, and LaTonya Noel, MSW, are both Doctoral Candidates; all affiliated with the University of Texas at Austin School of Social Work.

Address correspondence to: Elizabeth C. Pomeroy, PhD, LCSW, University of Texas at Austin School of Social Work, 1 University Station, D3500, Austin, TX 78712 (E-mail: Bpomeroy@mail.utexas.edu).

The authors would like to thank Tracy Kulik of Collaborative Research for her role in this project.

[Haworth co-indexing entry note]: "Predictors of Medication Adherence Among HIV/AIDS Clients." Pomeroy, Elizabeth C. et al. Co-published simultaneously in *the Journal of HIV/AIDS & Social Services* (The Haworth Press, Inc.) Vol. 6, No. 1/2, 2007, pp. 65-81; and: *HIV Treatment Adherence: Challenges for Social Services* (ed: Lana Sue Ka'opua and Nathan L. Linsk) The Haworth Press, Inc., 2007, pp. 65-81. Single or multiple copies of this article are available for a fee from The Haworth Document Delivery Service [1-800-HAWORTH, 9:00 a.m. - 5:00 p.m. (EST). E-mail address: docdelivery@haworthpress.com].

Available online at http://jhaso.haworthpress.com
© 2007 by The Haworth Press, Inc. All rights reserved.
doi: 10.1300/J187v06n01_05

This study seeks to identify factors that predict medication adherence among HIV positive adults. Independent variables included adherence information, adherence motivation, adherence behavioral skills, demographic factors and environmental factors. Results from the exploratory study using a convenience sample of patients lend support to Fisher's Information-Motivation-Behavior model of HIV prevention. Implications for research and practice are discussed. doi:10.1300/J187v06n01_05 *[Article copies available for a fee from The Haworth Document Delivery Service: 1-800-HAWORTH. E-mail address: <docdelivery@haworthpress.com> Website: <http://www.HaworthPress.com> © 2007 by The Haworth Press, Inc. All rights reserved.]*

KEYWORDS. HIV/AIDS, mental health services, medication adherence, compliance

INTRODUCTION

The introduction and success of antiretroviral medications has led to a remarkable decrease in HIV-related morbidity and mortality (Hogg et al., 1998; Palella et al., 1998). The various measures of HIV treatment, such as viral suppression and CD4 lymphocyte cell counts, are employed to reflect an individual's health status. New medication combinations have life-enhancing implications for individuals living with HIV infection. However, the regimens are complex, often requiring patients to take more than 24 pills throughout the day, at specific times, and with special instructions such as fasting and taking dose with high-fat meals (Chesney, Morin, & Sherr, 2000; Murphy, Roberts, & Martin, 2000). Although antiretroviral therapies have been found to be an effective in reducing the viral load in HIV positive patients; the characteristics of HAART medication regimens have been found to negatively impact medication adherence among HIV positive adults (Elred, Wu, Chaisson, & Moore, 1998; Paterson et al., 2000; Stone et al., 2001).

Lack of adherence to medication regimens among people living with HIV/AIDS contributes to the epidemic itself, as well as to the personal health of individual patients. From the patient's perspective, non-adherence to medications contributes to decreased CD4 counts (Manfredi, Calza, & Chiodo, 2001; Singh et al., 1999), increased viral load (Catz, Kelly, & Bogart, 2000; Knobel et al., 2002; Singh et al., 1999; Zaccarelli et al., 2002) and HIV-related mortality. Additionally, suboptimal adherence produces strains of the virus that are resistant to treatment in the original patient (Gallant, 2000; Tamalet et al., 2000).

These mutant strains of the virus can be transmitted to those already infected with HIV, as well as people who are HIV negative. Unfortunately, due to suboptimal adherence, the prevalence of these resistant strains continues to increase (Boden et al., 1999), posing a serious public health risk. Adherence to the various medications must be 95-100% complete in order to be considered adequate; however, 57% to 77% of patients fail to reach this level of adherence (Paterson et al., 2000; Spire, Duran, & Sourville, 2002). These patients run the risk of increased viral loads and the development of resistant strains of the virus for which no medications are available. In response to this risk, it has been reported that many doctors are reticent to give treatment to patients whom they believe are unlikely to comply with the treatment, such as homeless and drug-using individuals (Ickovics & Meade, 2002).

While Highly Active Antiretroviral Therapy (HAART) is effective in increasing incubation periods for those with HIV, this multi-drug therapy is intensive in terms of requirements on the patient. Side effects of these powerful drugs can be uncomfortable to the point of making patients violently ill (Ickovics & Meisler, 1997), and the regimen can be time consuming and awkward. The complexities of HAART treatment regimens may include several different medications with several daily doses, strict food and fluid dosing instructions and times of the day that the medications need to be taken. In addition, to these drugs that HIV positive patients take to reduce their viral load they may also take additional drugs to treat related ailments. Research suggests that these complicated regimens negatively impact HIV patients' medication adherence. In a study of 289 HIV infected patients, Stone et al. (2001), found that high regimen complexity was associated with decreased medication adherence. HAART medication schedules are also difficult to maintain, and can be especially problematic for the HIV population. Studies indicate that non-adherence rates among HIV positive patients on HAART range from 26% to 95% (Avants, Margolin, Warburton, Hawkins, & Shi, 2001; Aversa & Kimberlin, 1996; Ickovics & Meade, 2002; Spire et al., 2002). Medication and treatment issues related to medication compliance include sleeping through dose time, special instructions, change in daily routine, lack of medications away from home, didn't allow time to take medications, forgetfulness, avoiding side effects, and large numbers of pills (Murphy et al., 2000).

Other factors related to medication adherence are complex and have yet to be explored sufficiently. A meta-analysis of 29 studies between

1998 and 2002 was used to identify factors related to medication adherence (Ammassari, Trotta, & Murri, 2002). According to the researchers, medication/treatment issues and psychosocial factors are most consistently related to medication adherence. Although many behavioral issues and patient variables were not clearly or consistently related to medication compliance, most of these results are based on relatively small samples that lack the power to detect significance.

The purpose of this study is to identify factors that predict medication adherence among HIV positive adults. Independent variables to be studied include adherence information, adherence motivation, adherence behavioral skills, demographic factors and environmental factors. Adherence motivation will include indicators of motivation specifically related to medication adherence in HIV patients, but will also include measures of social support, behavioral intent, and religious involvement. Adherence information will include indicators directly related to the patient's knowledge of their medication. Adherence behavioral skills will include indicators of skills related to medication adherence. Social support will include indicators of family and friends who have knowledge of the person's HIV status. Figure 1 illustrates the factors and their potential prediction of the dependent variable, medication adherence. It is hypothesized that each of the factors will predict medication adherence among HIV positive patients.

The modified model above is based on Fisher's Information, Motivation, and Behavior (IMB) model (Fisher & Fisher, 1992). The information-motivation-behavioral skills (IMB) model provides the conceptual

FIGURE 1. IMB Model Modified for Medication Adherence

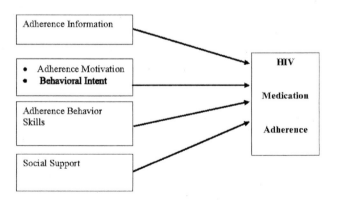

framework for the current study. It will be used to explore factors related to medication adherence. The model illustrates how obtaining prevention information, having motivation (including behavioral intent) to adhere to medication, and employing behavioral skills can lead to adherence behaviors (Fisher & Fisher, 1992, Fisher & Fisher, 1993). In addition, social support was added as a factor that could impact adherence behaviors. Theoretically, social supports are seen as instrumental in patient adaptation to illness and acceptance of treatment. There are two main theoretical positions which attempt to explain the relationship between medication adherence and social support. The first suggests that social support plays a significant role in buffering stress related to the adaptation to illness and the other suggests that social support is inherently important to all persons. Research also suggests that the presence or absence of social supports are consistent predictors of medication adherence in HIV/AIDS positive populations (Berg et al., 2004; Catz, Heckman, Kochman, & DiMarco, 2001; Garcia & Cote, 2003).

Fisher's model particularly focuses on information, motivation, and behavior skills as factors that lead to actual behavior. This model has been used to study prevention among HIV negative populations, such as adolescents (Fisher, Williams et al., 1998) and Indian truck drivers (Bryan, Fisher, & Benziger, 2001). It has also been used in relation to sexual risk behaviors (Fisher, Kimbele-Willcutts, Misovich, & Weinstein, 1997) and sharing needles (Fisher, Misovich et al., 1998) among the HIV positive population.

METHODS

Research Design

A confidential and anonymous survey was designed to collect information about the correlates and predictors of medication adherence in culturally distinct groups of Persons Living with HIV/AIDS (PLWH/A). The sample of approximately 225 individuals surveyed comprised a representative subset of the population of people living with HIV/AIDS (PLWH/A) in a large metropolitan area in central Texas. Using quota sampling techniques, the ethnic characteristics of survey subjects matched the ethnic characteristics of the county's population estimates as identified by the County Department of Health and the Centers for Disease Control and Prevention ([CDC], 2004, Texas Department of State Health Services, 2004). This technique was used in an attempt to obtain a representative sample of the region's population. Of the 225 original surveys completed, 41 surveys were eliminated due to incomplete information on key variables of interest; 184 (82%) surveys were utilized in the final analysis. Surveyed participants were over the age of 18, in various stages of health, ranging from asymptomatic to terminally ill with AIDS. All participants were ambulatory or able to be transported to public sites with routine assistance.

Surveys were conducted between June 1 and August 15, 2004 at community sites and agencies where respondents regularly received services. Trained research assistants administered the surveys after potential participants were screened by agency staff for competency to answer survey questions. Based on language preferences, some subjects completed the survey in Spanish. If a potential participant wanted to complete the survey, but lacked the literacy required to complete the survey, a survey administrator read the survey to the participant. The survey took approximately 60 minutes to complete.

Respondents were solicited through posting of flyers and word of mouth at eight HIV/AIDS organizations in the South-Central Texas area. Both in-care and out-of-care adults were encouraged to participate in the survey. Survey completion sessions were arranged by service agencies. Participation was voluntary and participants were compensated with merchandise vouchers provided by the HIV Planning Council in recognition of the time spent completing the survey.

Informed consent was obtained from each adult at the time of survey administration. Research assistants were available to review consent forms and respond to questions. A copy of the consent form was given to each of the survey participants. After survey data were collected, they were entered into a dataset with no identifying information (i.e., name, address) included.

Research Questions

The research questions of this study were as follows:

1. To what extent are HIV+ adults adherent to their medication and treatment regimen?
2. What is the relationship between medication adherence and intention-motivation-behavioral factors and medical service use among HIV+ adults?

3. To what extent do demographic and environmental predictors account for the difference in medication adherence among this sample of HIV+ adults?

Measures

The survey questions included basic demographic information, medication/treatment information, service utilization, and medication adherence. As delineated in Fischer's IMB model, the construct of "adherence" consists of adherence information, motivation, and behavioral factors. The authors of this study also utilized social support as an additional factor in order to examine its contribution to adherence (see Table 1). The medication adherence scale (Fischer & Fischer, 1992; 1993) and the Social Support and Reciprocity Scale (Hoppe, 1997) utilized in this study are described in the following paragraphs.

Medication Adherence Measures

Self-Reported Levels of Medication Adherence were determined by self-reported frequency of missed doses per week. Response choices coded 1-4, included: 1 = "Never," 2 = "Rarely (no more than once a week)," 3 = "Some of the time (one to four times a week)," and 4 = "Often (five or more times a week)" respectively.

Adherence Information was based on four questions. Response choices included: 0 = "Not Sure," 1 = "True," and 2 = "False." Questions were ·related to knowing what to do if a dose is missed, whether the respondent

TABLE 1. Adherence Measurement Criteria

Adherence Criteria	Mean	SD	Range of Measure	Range of Participant Scores
Adherence behavior skills*	20.73	5.3	0-30	3-30
Adherence information*	1.85	1.1	0-2	0-2
Motivation due to perceived vulnerability*	8.15	2.2	2-10	2-10
Motivation due to provider support*	11.89	4.1	1-15	1-15
Social normative support for adherence*	7.98	2.6	1-10	1-10
Intentions to adhere*	8.12	1.8	4-10	4-10

*Higher scores indicate higher levels of attribute measured

thought they could miss a few pills every once in a while without damaging their health, what the effect would be if non-prescription drugs were taken, and an understanding of the side effects of the combination of medications in their treatment.

Social Normative Support for Adherence was measured by two items related to whether friends and family think the respondent should comply with the medication regimen; response choices were based on a five-point scale ranging from 1 = Strongly Disagree to 5 = Strongly Agree.

Motivation Due to Provider Support was measured using the same five-point scale; three questions addressed the respondent's perception of help from their doctor, faith in their doctor, and belief that they are doing their best.

Motivation Due to Perceived Vulnerability was measured by two questions using a five-point scale ranging from 1 = Definitely Not to 5 = Definitely Yes. The questions addressed the respondent's belief that they will be able to control their HIV with the treatment, and their belief that the treatment will help them live longer.

Intentions to Adhere based on behavior questions ranged in response on a 5-point scale from 1 = "None of the Time" to 5 = "All of the Time." The questions related to whether the patient expected to adhere to the medication regimen in the next three months.

Adherence Behavior Skills were assessed through a series of six questions using a five-point scale ranging from 1 = Strongly Disagree to 5 = Strongly Agree. Questions were related to difficulty in taking medications appropriately due to not having the right food or liquid on hand, difficult remembering the regimen, no problems taking the medications correctly, taking the medications according to doctor's orders, taking the medications despite side effects, and confidence in gaining additional information if necessary.

Social Support and Reciprocity Scale (Hoppe, 1997) specifically assessed one's support in relation to their HIV status. This measure examines potential sources of support and the perceived likelihood of receiving help from each friend or family member that the respondent has included on a pre-established list on a five-point scale ranging from 1 = Strongly Disagree to 5 = Strongly Agree.

These scales have been utilized in several studies as noted above and are found to be reliable indicators of the variable under study. However, psychometric properties of these scales are still in the developmental stage; therefore, the scales have not been standardized nor have cut points been identified to designate high, medium, and low levels of each phenomenon.

Data Analysis

Data analyses began with an examination of the characteristics of individual variables and simple relationships between variables; this examination was completed prior to conducting more complex multivariate analyses. Initial descriptive analyses, such as frequency distributions, were used to analyze demographic data (see Table 2). Means, standard deviations, proportions and the standard errors of interval data and confidence limits of major variables of interest were calculated to provide complete descriptions of their distributions. These preliminary examinations were necessary to interpret more complex multivariate analyses.

Following the univariate analyses, single-order correlations were conducted to determine relationships between medication adherence and adherence information, motivation, behavioral skills, social support and other demographic variables. Collinearity diagnostics showed tolerances between .7-.9; each predictor variable was determined to be a separate factor and appropriate for simultaneous inclusion in regression models. Ordinary Least Squares multiple regression analyses were conducted to examine the joint relationship between the dependent variable, adherence, and two or more independent predictor variables such as motivation, ethnicity, and/or behavioral intentions. Multiple regression coefficients (β) measure the amount of increase in adherence for a

TABLE 2. Multiple Regression Models to Predict Adherence

Predictors	Full sample		Caucasian		Latino	
	β	(p value)	β	(p value)	β	(p value)
Number of children in household	.06	.44	.10	.43	.21	.10
Received medical care within 1 year of diagnosis	.18	.02*	.28	.03*	.51	.01*
Currently receiving mental health services	.14	.06	.03	.81	.06	.63
Received adherence information	.22	.01*	.42	.01*	.31	.03*
Motivation due to perceived vulnerability	.20	.02*	.21	.14	.05	.73
Motivation due to provider	.01	.92	.05	.75	.04	.76
Social support for adherence	.09	.29	.02	.90	.07	.57
Intention to adhere	.21	.01*	.24	.07	.19	.17
Variance explained	$R^2 = .36$		$R^2 = .29$		$R^2 = .47$	

* $p \leq .05$

one-unit difference in each independent variable, controlling for the other independent variables. Only those variables significantly associated with medication adherence on a bivariate level were included in the regression analyses.

RESULTS

The sample ($N = 184$) consisted primarily of males ($N = 157, 78\%$) and females ($N = 28, 15\%$), but fourteen subjects (7%) self-identified as "transgender." They averaged 43 years of age (M = 43.2, SD = 7.3) and were predominantly Hispanic ($N = 72, 39\%$), White ($N = 64, 35\%$), or African American ($N = 31, 17\%$). Native American, Asians and other ethnicities accounted for the remaining 9 percent ($N = 17$) of the sample. Most respondents reported attending some high school ($N = 53, 29\%$) or completing high school ($N = 44, 24\%$); however, many had some college or advanced education ($N = 88, 48\%$). The majority of respondents identified themselves as single ($N = 77, 42\%$), partnered ($N = 33, 18\%$), or divorced ($N = 37, 20\%$). Married/common law and widowed participants comprised 20 percent ($N = 37$) of the sample; few ($N = 32, 17\%$) had children living in their household. The majority reported they believed they had been infected with HIV due to having sex with men ($N = 118, 64\%$), whereas only 15% ($N = 28$) believed they had become infected through sharing needles. Finally, most participants ($N = 146, 79\%$) were currently receiving HIV services.

The first research question addressed the extent to which HIV positive adults were adherent to their medication and treatment regimen. The majority of participants ($N = 131, 71\%$) reported they had little to no difficulty taking their combination therapy medications. In addition, results from the Fisher and Fisher (1992, 1993) medication adherence scale, which measures adherence behaviors and other factors, indicated that the majority of respondents were moderately adherent with the antiretroviral regimen (mean = 20.7, SD = 5.3, range 3-30). While no cut point is identified by this scale's authors, higher scores indicate greater adherence. As scores range from 0-30, the mean score of 20.7 suggests that most individuals were moderately adherent.

The second research question sought to evaluate the relationship between medication adherence, the factors of the IMB model, and medical service use among HIV positive adults. Results on the medication adherence scale indicated that HIV positive respondents identified adherence information, motivation due to perceived vulnerability and provider support as being significant factors associated with medication adherence. The following variables were significantly associated with greater medication adherence: fewer children in the household ($r = -.16$, $p < .04$), receiving medical care within the first year of HIV diagnosis ($r = .24, p < .004$), currently receiving mental health services ($r = .24$, $p < .003$), receiving adherence information ($r = .42, p < .0001$), increased motivation to comply with medication regimens due to the individual's perceived vulnerability ($r = .40, p < .0001$), increased motivation due to provider relationship ($r = .29., p < .0001$), increased social support from family and peers ($r = .32, p < .0001$), and intentions to adhere ($r = .40, p < .0001$). Demographics, such as gender, age, ethnicity, marital status, and education, were not associated with adherence.

The final research question assessed the extent to which the predictor variables account for medication adherence. A multivariate analysis was performed using only those variables, which the bivariate analysis detected as significantly associated with adherence. Similar analyses were then conducted to test predictors for white and Latino participants only. The multiple regression model for the entire sample, as shown in Table 2, indicated that getting medical care within the first year of being diagnosed with HIV, receiving information about adherence issues, being motivated to adhere due to feelings of perceived vulnerability, and intentions to adhere to treatment were significant ($p < .05$) predictors of increased medication adherence ($F[8, 124] = 8.82, p < .001$). This model accounted for 36 percent of the variance explained in medication adherence.

In the regression model of white participants only, the analysis showed that getting medical care within the first year of being diagnosed with HIV, receiving information about adherence issues and intending to adhere to treatment were significant ($p < .10$) predictors of increased adherence ($F[8, 41] = 3.55, p < .003$) and explained 29% of the variance in adherence. Among Latinos, regression analyses indicated that having more children, getting medical care within the first year of HIV diagnosis, and receiving information about adherence issues significantly predicted greater adherence ($F[8, 43] = 6.69, p < .001$). This model explained 47 percent of the variance in medication adherence.

DISCUSSION

The results of this study provide further validation for the use of Fischer's IMB model for understanding medication adherence among HIV positive adults. First, HIV positive respondents stated that adherence information was a significant factor in their ability to adhere to HIV medications despite the difficult regimens. Secondly, respondents indicated that motivation due to perceived vulnerability and provider support were necessary prerequisites to controlling their illness through consistent medication use. In addition, respondents' intentions to adhere were a significant predictor to actual adherence behaviors. The researchers examined social support in relation to medication adherence and found that supportive peers and family members were a key component to the medication adherence process. They further modified the model to include mental health service utilization that was also found to be a factor in medication adherence. Finally, following recommendations for taking medications included: having food and liquids on hand, remembering the regimen accurately, following physician's medication directions, consistently taking medications despite side effects, and receiving clarification from medical staff about medications. These behavioral skills appear to predict medication adherence in this sample of HIV positive adults.

Results indicated that some cultural differences existed among participants of this pilot study. While results indicated that having more children in the household led to greater adherence among Latinos, this finding may not be unique to this population. Only 17.4% ($N = 32$) of participants had children and the majority of these respondents were Latino, therefore; these results may reflect the lack of random selection. While having more children in the home is an important predictor of adherence for Latinos, the lack of representation of other ethnic groups with children in this sample prevents any comparative conclusions. On the other hand, researchers may want to examine this variable in future studies in order to assess if this predictor varies or remains the same across ethnic groups.

For both Latino and Caucasian participants, getting medical care during the first year after diagnosis and receiving information about adherence were important predictors of adherence to medication. This finding may suggest that these services are important for HIV positive persons in general, although more research is needed on the impact of these services on other ethnic groups.

In summary, our findings indicate that the combination of the following factors predict 36% of the variance in medication adherence: receiving medical care within one year of diagnosis, currently receiving mental health services, receiving adherence information, motivation due to perceived vulnerability and intentions to adhere. Further research is needed to examine other factors that may contribute to HIV positive patients' abilities to adhere to medication regimens.

Limitations

While the current findings uphold Fischer's IMB model, the results should be viewed with caution, because this was a pilot study utilizing a small sample from one urban area. A larger sample using random sampling could lead to increased generalizability of results. The quota sampling methods employed for this study may have resulted in inherent biases, particularly when the method is based on ethnicity alone (Rubin & Babbie, 1997). In the southern part of the U.S. where this study was conducted, the population was predominantly Caucasian and Latino with an under-representation of African Americans and other ethnic groups. This lack of diversity limited the scope of this study in terms of examining ethnic differences. A more extensive examination of ethnicity in terms of medication adherence is an important area of research with regard to cultural competence in working with diverse client groups. Secondly, participants were volunteers recruited for the study. Therefore, individuals who did not hear about the study or who were not involved in an AIDS organization would not have participated in this study. In addition, there may have been unique characteristics among the 18% ($N = 33$) of respondents whom were dropped from the analysis due to incomplete surveys, which may have affected the results.

Implications for Social Work Research and Practice

Despite the limitations discussed, the study provides valuable insights into how clients adhere to difficult and complicated medication regimens. When clients receive information concerning the importance of medication adherence, they are more likely to follow a complicated medication regimen. From a clinical perspective, clients need information that is clear, concise and understandable. It may also be important to provide information in both verbal and written format. It would be helpful for clients to obtain this information in their primary, spoken language and at a level that is easily comprehended. Laminated handouts that highlight the dosing schedules for each medication would help clients learn and follow the prescribed regimen. Follow-up information sessions with a doctor or allied health professional would allow clients to ask questions and clarify any misconceptions about the reading material or medication regimen.

Increased motivation due to the client's relationship with the provider and perceived vulnerability are key factors in medication adherence. In a qualitative study of HIV positive adults (Haney, Pomeroy & Noel, 2004), participants reported that having a trusting, working relationship with their primary care physician influenced their attitude toward taking medications on a daily, routine basis. Due to the chronic and stigmatized nature of the illness, having a long-term relationship with a physician allows for greater trust and thus greater compliance with the physician's recommendations.

An increased self-efficacy to manage the medications regardless of bio-psycho-social effects is lead by the open dialogue between friends, family members and the HIV positive adult about the illness and the medication regimens. Mental health services also appear to provide additional support to clients on retroviral therapies. Social workers may facilitate services for clients. This may include working with clients' families and friends to understand the illness and provide emotional support. It has been shown that clients with a network of support have better physical and mental health outcomes. Social workers can play a pivotal role in providing clients with these valuable services.

CONCLUSION

Future research regarding medication adherence should focus on examining potential differences by gender and ethnicity. From the qualitative study conducted by some of the researchers (Haney et al., 2004), it was clear that men and women encountered unique obstacles and used different techniques to remain compliant to their medication protocols. In the same study, the three identified ethnic groups (African American, Hispanic and Caucasian) offered distinct perceptions about coping with complicated medication schedules. This suggests the need for future research to explore these factors in more detail.

Finally, research regarding best practices for engaging HIV positive adults who are not receiving medical services is needed to encourage treatment initiation. This is a major public health issue because HIV positive adults who are not receiving medical attention are at increased risk of spreading the illness to others, as well as contracting opportunistic infections themselves. In addition, research in the area of incorporating mental health interventions into primary care clinics that serve HIV positive clients could support clients and physicians in managing medications and mental health concerns. In summary, as HIV becomes a more long term, chronic condition that mandates medication for control of the disease, clients will continually need to acquire new information and coping techniques. Rather than preparing for a terminal condition, HIV positive adults are now accessing a wide variety of services in order to manage their illness and maintain their health. Social service providers can provide timely information about HAART and adherence to newly diagnosed clients so that linkages to early medical care can be made. By receiving this information in a timely manner, clients can be assured better health outcomes and quality of life. In addition, social service providers can assist family members by providing accurate information about medication adherence who can, in turn, assist the HIV positive individual with their health care needs.

REFERENCES

Ammassari, A., Trotta, M. P., Murri, R., Castelli, F., Narciso, P., Noto, P. et al. (2002). Correlates and predictors of adherence to highly active antiretroviral therapy: Overview of published literature. *Journal of Acquired Immune Deficiency Syndromes, 31*, S123-S127.

Avants, S. K., Margolin, A., Warburton, L. A., Hawkins, K. A., & Shi, J. (2001). Predictors of nonadherence to HIV-related medication regimens during methadone stabilization. *The American Journal of Addictions, 10*, 69-78.

Aversa, S. L., & Kimberlin, C. (1996). Psychosocial aspects of antiretroviral medication use among HIV patients. *Patient Education and Counseling, 29*, 207-219.

Berg, K. M., Demas, P. A., Howard, A. A., Schoenbaum, E. E., Gourevitch, M. N., & Arnsen, J. H. (2004). Gender differences in factors associated with adherence to antiretroviral therapy. *Journal of General Internal Medicine, 19*, 1111-1117.

Boden, D., Hurley, A., Zhang, L., Cao, Y., Guo, Y., & Jones, E. et al. (1999). HIV-1 drug resistance in newly infected individuals. *Journal of the American Medical Association, 282*, 1135-1141.

Bryan, A. D., Fisher, J. D., & Benziger, T. J. (2001). Determinants of HIV risk among Indian truck drivers. *Social Science & Medicine, 53*(11), 1413-1426.

Catz, S. L., Heckman, T. G., Kochman, A., & DiMarco, M. (2001). Rates and correlates of HIV treatment adherence among late middle-aged and older adults living with HIV disease. *Psychology of Health and Medicine, 6*, 47-58.

Catz, S. L., Kelly, J. A., & Bogart, L. M. (2000). Patterns, correlates, and barriers to medication adherence among persons prescribed new treatments for HIV disease. *Health Psychology, 19(2)*, 124-133.

Chesney, M. A., Morin, M., & Sherr, L. (2000). Adherence to HIV combination therapy. *Social Science and Medicine, 50*, 1599-1605.

Eldred, L. J., Wu, A. W., Chaisson, R. E., & Moore, R. D. (1998). Adherence to antiretroviral and pneumocystis prophylaxis in HIV disease. *Journal of Acquired Immune Deficiency Syndrome and Human Retrovirology, 18*, 117-125.

Fisher, J. D., & Fisher, W. (1992). Changing AIDS risk behavior. *Psychological Bulletin, 111*, 455-474.

Fisher, W. A., & Fisher, J. D. (1993). A general social psychological model for changing AIDS risk behavior. In J. B. Pryor & G. D. Reeder (Eds.), *The social psychology of HIV infection* (pp. 127-153). Hillsdale, NJ: Erlbaum.

Fisher, J. D., Kimble-Willcutts, D. L., Misovich, S. J., & Weinstein, B. (1997). Dynamics of sexual risk behavior in HIV-infected men who have sex with men. *AIDS and Behavior, 2*(2), 101-113.

Fisher, J. D., Misovich, S. J., Kimble, D. L., & Weinstein, B. (1998). Dynamics of HIV risk behavior in HIV-infected injection drug users. *AIDS and Behavior, 3*, 41-57.

Fisher, W. A., Williams, S. S., Fisher, J. D., & Malloy, T. E. (1998). Understanding AIDS risk behavior among sexually active urban adolescents: An empirical test of the Information-Motivation-Behavioral Skills Model. *AIDS and Behavior, 3*(1), 13-23.

Gallant, J. E. (2000). Strategies for long-term success in the treatment of HIV infection. *Journal of the American Medical Association, 283*, 1329-1334.

Garcia, P. R., & Cote, J. K. (2003). Factors affecting adherence to antiretroviral therapy in people living with HIV/AIDS. *Journal of the Association of Nurses in AIDS Care, 14*, 37-45.

Haney, M., Pomeroy, E. C., & Noel, L. (2004). Medication adherence among HIV positive clients: A pilot study. Unpublished manuscript.

Hogg, R., Rhone, S. A., Yip, B., Sherlock, C., Conway, B., Schechter, M. T. et al. (1998). Antiretroviral effect of double and triple drug combinations among HIV-infected adults: Lessons learned from the implementation of viral-load driven antiretroviral therapy. *AIDS, 12*, 279-284.

Hoppe, S. (1997). A measure of disclosure to network members. Unpublished manuscript, University of Texas Health Science Center at San Antonio.

Ickovics, J. R., & Meade, C. S. (2002). Adherence to antiretroviral therapy among patients with HIV: A critical link between behavioral and biomedical sciences. *Journal of Acquired Immune Deficiency Syndromes, 31*, S98-S102.

Ickovics, J. R., & Meisler, A. W. (1997). Adherence in AIDS clinical trials: A framework for clinical research and clinical care. *Journal of Clinical Epidemiology, 50*, 385-391.

Knobel, H., Alonso, J., Casado, J. L., Collazos, J., Gonzalez, J., Ruiz, I. et al. (2002). Validation of a simplified medication adherence questionnaire in a large cohort of HIV-infected patients: The GEEMA Study. *AIDS, 16*(4), 605-13.

Manfredi, R., Calza, L., & Chiodo, F. (2001). Dual nucleoside analogue treatment in the era of highly active antiretroviral therapy (HAART): A single-centre cross-sectional survey. *The Journal of Antimicrobial Chemotherapy, 48*(2), 299-302.

Murphy, D. A., Roberts, K. J., & Martin, D. J. (2000). Barriers to antiretroviral adherence among HIV-infected adults. *AIDS Patient Care & STD's, 14*(1), 47-58.

Murphy, D. A., Wilson, C. M., Durako, S. J., Muenz, L. R., Belzer, M., Friedman, L. et al. (2001). Antiretrovial medication adherence among the REACH HIV-infected adolescent cohort in the USA. *AIDS Care, 13*, 27-40.

Palella, F. J., Delaney, K. M., Moorman, A. C., Loveless, M. O., Fuhrer, J., Satten, G. A. et al. (1998). Declining morbidity and mortality among patients with advanced human immunodeficiency virus infection: HIV outpatient study investigators. *New England Journal of Medicine, 338*, 853-860.

Paterson, D., Swindells, S., Mohr, J., Brester, M., Vergis, E., Squier, C. et al. (2000). Adherence to protease inhibitor therapy and outcomes in patients with HIV infections. *Annals of Internal Medicine, 133*, 21-30.

Rubin, A., & Babbie, E. (1997). *Research methods for social work* (3rd Ed.). Pacific Grove: Wadsworth Publishing.

Singh, N., Berman, S. M., Swindells, S., Justis, J. C., Mohr, J. A., Squier, C. et al. (1999). Adherence of human immunodeficiency virus-infected patients to antiretroviral therapy. *Clinical Infectious Diseases, 29*, 824-830.

Spire, B., Duran, S., & Sourville, M. (2002). Adherence to highly active antiretroviral therapies (HAART) in HIV-infected patients: From a predictive to a dynamic approach. *Social Science & Medicine, 54(10)*, 1481-1496.

Stone, V. E., Hogan J. W., Schuman, P., Rompalo, A. M., Howard, A. A., Korkontzelou, C. et al. (2001). Antiretroviral regimen complexity, self-reported adherence, and HIV patients' understanding of their regimens: Survey of women in the HER study. *Journal of Acquired Immune Deficiency Syndrome, 28*(2), 124-131.

Tamalet, C., Pasquier, C., Yahi, N., Colson, P., Poizot-Martin, I., Lepu, G. et al. (2000). Prevalence of drug resistant mutants and virological response to combination therapy in patients with primary HIV-1 infection. *Journal of Medical Virology, 61*(2), 181-186.

Zaccarelli, M., Barracchini, A., De Longis, P., Perno, C. F., Soldani, F., Liuzzi, G. et al. (2002). Factors related to virologic failure among HIV-positive injecting drug users treated with combination antiretroviral therapy including two nucleoside reverse transcriptase inhibitors and nevirapine. *AIDS Patient Care and STDs, 16*, 67-73.

doi:10.1300/J187v06n01_05

Social and Religious Support
on Treatment Adherence Among
HIV/AIDS Patients by Race/Ethnicity

T. S. Sunil, PhD, MPH
Mary A. McGehee, PhD

SUMMARY. Using data from the second follow-up of the HIV Cost and Services Utilization Study (HCSUS), we investigated the influence of social and religious support variables on treatment adherence for Whites, African American and Hispanic HIV patients. Study results show differential effects of social, religious support and background variables on treatment adherence. In general, for Whites, background variables such as educational levels and age were found to be significant variables affecting treatment adherence, in addition to some religious support variables. On the other hand, for African Americans and Hispanics,

---

T. S. Sunil, PhD, MPH, is Assistant Professor in the Department of Sociology at University of Texas at San Antonio.

Mary A. McGehee, PhD, is Senior Research Analyst in the Center for Health Statistics, Arkansas Department of Health and Human Services.

Address correspondence to: T. S. Sunil, University of Texas, Department of Sociology, 6900 North Loop 1604 West, San Antonio, TX 78249 (E-mail: thankam.sunil@utsa.edu).

The authors thank the Agency for Healthcare Research and Quality, Rockville, MD, for sharing their HCSUS database. Comments from the journal's anonymous reviewers were extremely helpful in finalizing the paper.

[Haworth co-indexing entry note]: "Social and Religious Support on Treatment Adherence Among HIV/ AIDS Patients by Race/Ethnicity." Sunil, T.S., and Mary A. McGehee. Co-published simultaneously in *the Journal of HIV/AIDS & Social Services* (The Haworth Press, Inc.) Vol. 6, No. 1/2, 2007, pp. 83-99; and: *HIV Treatment Adherence: Challenges for Social Services* (ed: Lana Sue Ka'opua and Nathan L. Linsk) The Haworth Press, Inc., 2007, pp. 83-99. Single or multiple copies of this article are available for a fee from The Haworth Document Delivery Service [1-800-HAWORTH, 9:00 a.m. - 5:00 p.m. (EST). E-mail address: docdelivery@haworthpress.com].

Available online at http://jhaso.haworthpress.com
doi: 10.1300/J187v06n01_06

religious and social support variables were influential. Results also suggest that strategies to improve treatment adherence may vary for different race/ethnic groups. The study highlights the importance of working with and involving religious organizations in an effort to increase adherence and support to HIV-infected members, particularly among African Americans and Hispanic communities. doi:10.1300/J187v06n01_06 *[Article copies available for a fee from The Haworth Document Delivery Service: 1-800-HAWORTH. E-mail address: <docdelivery@haworthpress.com> Website: <http:// www.HaworthPress.com> © 2007 by The Haworth Press, Inc. All rights reserved.]*

KEYWORDS. HIV/AIDS, social support, religious support, treatment adherence, race/ethnicity

INTRODUCTION

Adherence to treatment medications is important to decrease morbidity and mortality related to any illness, including the human immunodeficiency virus (HIV). It is of utmost importance to patients living with HIV, since antiretroviral medications suppress the HIV viral load to undetectable levels and improve CD4 counts (Golin et al., 2002; Meichenbaum & Turk, 1987; Shapiro, Berk et al., 1999). Additionally, several studies have shown that in order to control any development of drug-resistant viral strains, HIV patients must adhere to 90-95 percent of the prescribed doses of medication (Paterson et al., 2000; Bangsberg et al., 2001). This level of adherence is especially difficult to maintain considering the complexity of the treatment regimen (Palella et al., 1998; Wright, 2000).

A number of studies have indicated that social support, which includes emotional, instrumental, and appraisal support, has a positive relationship with treatment adherence among HIV patients (Berkman, Glass, Brissette, & Seeman, 2000; Catz, Kelly, Bogart, Benotsch, & McAuliffe, 2000; Catz, McClure, Jones, & Brantley, 1999; Power et al, 2003.; Schwarzer, Dunkel-Schetter, & Kemeny, 1994; Shapiro, Morton et al., 1999) because of its buffering effect on problems such as hopelessness, psychological distress, and low-perceived self-efficacy can be deterrents to adherence (Blythe, 1983; Tucker, Burnam, Sherbourne, Kung, & Gifford, 2003; Williams & Friedland, 1997; Berkman et al.). However, at least two major limitations can be found in these studies. First, the studies do not incorporate variables measuring religious or spiritual support as a source of social support in their analytical models. Second, these studies usually fail to analyze the difference in the influence of different types of social support on treatment adherence by race and ethnicity. Studies that do include an analysis by race and ethnicity usually compare results for Whites and African Americans and exclude the Hispanic population (Gant & Ostrow, 1995; Heckman et al., 2000). Given the fact that the Hispanic population is both rapidly increasing and disproportionately affected by HIV, it is important to include this population group in analyses (Centers for Disease Control and Prevention [CDC], 2002). The purpose of this study is to investigate the influence of both social and religious support variables on treatment adherence for White, African American, and Hispanic HIV patients using secondary data from the second follow-up of the HIV Cost and Services Utilization Study (HCSUS). Specifically, we are addressing two research questions. First, does religious support have any impact on treatment adherence for persons with HIV/AIDS? Second, does the influence of social and religious support vary by race/ethnicity? We hypothesize that religious support, as well as social support will be beneficial to treatment adherence for all three populations with religious support being especially beneficial for African Americans.

LITERATURE REVIEW

Religion and Spirituality

In this study, we use the concepts of religion (religiousness, religiosity) and spirituality as related, interchangeable constructs. Doing so requires some clarification and explanation because there have been attempts to polarize the definitions of religion and spirituality and to use them as separate constructs. Religion is often viewed as being an institutional construct, concerned mainly with doctrinal practices and organized, formal worship. However, religion or religiousness can also be conceptualized at the individual level, as when people refer to themselves as being religious, meaning that they tend to follow some set of beliefs or practices (James, 1961). Spirituality is considered to be more personal, representing a search or process through which individuals seek to discover, hold on to, or transform whatever is sacred in their lives (Pargament, 1997). The polarization of these constructs ignores two important facts. First, spirituality usually takes place in either a traditional or nontraditional religious context, so people often do not make a distinction between the two concepts. Second, a focus of these traditional religious organizations is helping people to improve their lives, which is also a basis for spirituality (Hill et al., 2000; Wunthnow, 1998). Church membership and attendance have been found to be strongly associated with spirituality (Simoni, Martone, & Kerwin, 2002). Because of the close relationship between religion and spirituality, a number of studies examining the effects of religion and spirituality on health have used these terms either interchangeably or as the same construct (Avants, Warburton, & Margolin, 2001; Hill & Pargament, 2003). They are treated as such in this study.

A number of pathways through which religious or spiritual support benefits the health or well-being of persons with chronic and life-threatening diseases, including those with HIV/AIDS have been suggested. First, the religious support that individuals receive from their church members, leaders, and clergy may help enhance self-esteem, be valuable as a source of information and companionship, and provide aid that can help buffer the effects of stress (Cohen & Wills, 1985). Religious support is associated with reducing adult mortality (Rogers, 1996; Rogers, Hummer, & Nam, 2000; Zuckerman, Kasl, & Ostfeld, 1984) and depression (Williams, Larson, Buckler, Heckman, & Pyle, 1991), as well as facilitating addiction recovery among HIV positive injection drug users (Avants et al., 2001); however, the influence of religious support has yet to be investigated in the critical area of treatment adherence to Highly Active Antiretroviral Therapy (HAART).

Second, spirituality may provide a sense of meaning and hope to persons threatened with an end to their existence (Mullen, Smith, & Hill, 1993; Pargament & Hahn, 1986). The difficulties of living with a life-threatening disease can cause people to rely more on their spirituality. Increased spirituality, for example, is a common response to being HIV positive (Jones, Catz, McClure, Jeffries, & Baglio, 1996). Spirituality also enhances one's coping abilities, and helps develop a positive attitude (Hall, 1994; Pargament, 1990). Jones et al., for example, found that prayer is a common coping strategy for persons of low socioeconomic status who have HIV. All these factors have been found to be related to treatment adherence (Blythe, 1983; Hall; Williams & Friedland, 1997).

Race/Ethnicity and Social Support

Studies focusing on race and ethnicity are important for a number of reasons. First, in addition to being disproportionately affected by HIV/AIDS (CDC, 2002), Hispanics and African Americans are more likely than their White counterparts to be faced with issues such as extreme homophobia, the effects of racism, culturally-based negative attitudes towards HIV infection, isolation, and low socioeconomic status that may be obstacles to their receiving social support (Dalton, 1989; Diaz, 1998; Siegel & Raveis, 1997). Further, the influence of different types of social support may vary by race and ethnicity (Ajouch, Antonucci, & Janevic, 2001). Research has indicated, for example, that African Americans and Whites differ in their use and source of formal and informal social support systems (Broman, 1987; Heckman et al., 2000; Neighbors & Jackson, 1987; Snowden, 1998). Heckman et al. found that older African American males with HIV were more likely to receive social support from family members while their white counterparts were more likely to receive support from friends. Also, religion and the church are important sources of social support for African Americans (Du Bois, 2000; Krause, 2002; Krause, 2003). Krause's research found that older African Americans are more religious than older whites and also attend church more. These research findings indicate that it is important to understand the impact of culture on social support for Hispanic and African American HIV/AIDS patients and the differences in the influences of various types of social support on treatment adherence by race and ethnicity.

METHODS

Data for the present study come from the HIV Cost and Services Utilization Study (HCSUS) conducted during 1997-1998. This survey is the first major research conducted from a nationally representative sample of HIV-infected adults in treatment and living in the United States (Frankel et al., 1999; Shapiro, Berk et al., 1999). The sample respondents were selected from 28 urban areas and 24 clusters of rural counties in the continental United States. The data for the background variables are from the baseline survey conducted from January 1996 to March 1997 (n = 2864), and the other variables are from the second follow-up, which was conducted from August 1997 to January 1998 (n = 2267). Details on sampling procedure and data collection maybe found elsewhere (Frankel et al., 1999; Shapiro, Berk et al., 1999; Tucker et al., 2003).

Dependent Variable

The dependent variable is derived from responses to questions on patients' antiretroviral medications. Fourteen different antiretroviral medications were identified in the survey. For each medication listed, four follow-up questions were asked: "Over the past week, how many days did you forget to take a dose of HIV medication?"; "Over the past week, how many days did you purposely not take a dose of HIV medication?"; How many days did you take a lesser amount than the prescribed dose of HIV medication?"; and "Over the past week, how many days did you take HIV medication exactly as your doctor prescribed you to take it?" We defined patients who took all medications exactly as prescribed in the past week as "adherent" and patients who missed one medication in the past week as "nonadherent." Following this definition, we found 888 adherent patients and 1022 nonadherent patients. Our dependent variable is dichotomous with nonadherent patients being coded 0 and adherent patients coded 1.

Independent Variables

Respondents were asked several questions on self-perceived social and religious support. The questions on social support indicate different types of support, namely, assistance and companionship. In addition to social and religious support variables, the following background characteristics were included: gender, ethnicity, age (18-34; 35-49; 50 and older) and educational level (some high school, no degree; high school degree; some college; BA, BS).

Associations between each of the independent variables and treatment adherence are analyzed both in the total patient cohort and within each of three racial/ethnic groups. Since the dependent variable is dichotomous, logistic regression is performed at the multivariate level. Separate logistic regressions were carried out for all the three racial/ethnic groups. Logistic regression is a type of regression analysis where the dependent variable is a dichotomous variable (say, coded 0 or 1). The effects of the independent variables are expressed in terms of odds ratios. That is, the ratio that something is true divided by the probability that it is not true. When odds are greater than 1, the event is more likely to happen than not (Mertler & Vannatta, 2004). Results reported here are based on analytical weights as recommended in the sampling description (Shapiro, Berk et al., 1999). Statistical weights are generally used in analysis to represent the survey data to the study population thus making results more generalizable.

RESULTS

Correlates of Adherence

There were 1910 patients taking antiretroviral medications in the second follow-up survey at the time of the data collection. Of the 1910 patients, 1022 patients (53.5 percent) were nonadherent and 888 (46.5 percent) were adherent to medications. Overall, patients who were adherent were more likely than those who were nonadherent to be White, male, older (50 and over), highly educated, less religious, to have someone to help them with daily chores, love them, and to give them money "all of the time." A bivariate distribution of all variables with status of treatment adherence was found to be statistically significant.

Adherence and Ethnicity

Table 1 allows us to examine any differences or similarities in characteristics of adherent and nonadherent patients by race/ethnicity. It shows treatment adherence status among different ethnic groups according to social support and religious support variables.

Two salient points are worth noting. First, religiosity varied more by race/ethnicity than by treatment adherence. That is, African Americans and Hispanics were much more likely than Whites to consider themselves to be religious, to attend religious services one or more times a month, or to seek comfort through religion. Second, for social support, the greatest differences in characteristics appear to be between adherent and nonadherent persons, particularly for African Americans. A higher percentage of adherent than nonadherent White, African American, and Hispanic patients had help with daily chores "all of the time." Also, for Whites, African Americans and Hispanics, adherent patients were more likely to have someone to love or someone to give them money "most of the time" or "all of the time." The greatest disparity in level of support between adherent and nonadherent patients for all three social support variables was for African Americans. For example, about 56 percent of the adherent African Americans compared to 41 percent of the nonadherent had someone to give them money most or all of the time. The corresponding percentages for Whites and Hispanics were 63.3 percent and 58.4 percent and 48.7 percent and 51.8 percent, respectively.

Adherence and Religious and Social Support

Results from the multivariate logistic regression are presented in Table 2.

As shown in this table, females of either racial/ethnic population had lower odds of adherence to antiretroviral medications than their male

TABLE 1. Percentage Distribution of Variables According to Race/Ethnicity and Adherence Status

Variables	Whites (N = 992)		African American (n = 581)		Hispanic (n = 272)	
	Nonadherent (n = 483)	Adherent (n = 509)	Nonadherent (n = 336)	Adherent (n = 245)	Nonadherent (n = 166)	Adherent (n = 106)
How religious are you?						
Not at all	17.4	19.8	4.0	6.0	10.1	14.9
Not very	22.9	24.9	10.3	11.2	21.5	12.0
Somewhat	41.9	40.7	43.9	40.4	50.2	44.8
Very	17.9	14.6	41.8	42.4	18.2	28.3
Religious attendance						
Never	39.7	47.3	18.7	19.3	30.0	41.3
Less than once a month	29.0	28.2	24.5	25.9	26.6	22.4
1-3 times a month	13.4	10.0	20.8	20.7	18.7	9.7
About once a week	10.2	9.4	20.6	21.1	16.9	13.6
More than once a week	7.7	5.1	15.5	12.9	7.7	13.0
Seek comfort through religion						
Never	21.5	26.9	7.7	6.7	17.4	10.8
Rarely	15.1	12.1	6.1	7.3	10.8	9.1
Sometimes	24.4	25.6	27.1	26.9	31.1	33.9
Often	39.0	35.4	59.1	59.2	40.7	46.2
Help with daily chores						
None of the time	9.3	9.6	15.3	13.1	14.3	14.2
A little of the time	12.4	7.2	9.7	4.1	8.8	3.8
Some of the time	9.8	8.9	16.5	13.4	11.2	12.7
Most of the time	25.2	22.8	21.4	19.9	28.3	14.8
All of the time	43.3	51.4	37.0	49.4	37.3	54.6
Someone to love						
None of the time	4.9	4.7	6.8	3.8	4.9	5.2
A little of the time	7.6	4.4	7.6	4.4	6.9	8.4
Some of the time	15.5	10.9	18.7	13.6	13.3	12.6
Most of the time	23.7	22.0	19.8	18.1	25.9	18.0
All of the time	48.3	58.0	47.1	60.2	49.0	55.8
Someone to give you money						
None of the time	15.0	14.5	20.1	13.7	16.6	22.2
A little of the time	14.0	8.9	15.8	14.2	11.1	8.3
Some of the time	12.6	13.2	23.1	16.2	20.5	20.8
Most of the time	18.7	19.6	18.3	11.7	21.6	16.5
All of the time	39.7	43.7	22.7	44.1	30.2	32.2

Note: 28 adherent patients and 37 nonadherent patients that reported "other" race are not included.

TABLE 2. Logistic Regression for Treatment Adherence

Variables	White Exp(B)	White 95% C.I.	African American Exp(B)	African American 95% C.I.	Hispanic Exp(B)	Hispanic 95% C.I.
Gender						
Male	1.00		1.00		1.00	
Female	0.79**	0.758-0.828	0.85**	0.813-0.879	0.66**	0.611-0.703
Age						
18-34	1.00		1.00		1.00	
35-49	1.08**	1.051-1.119	0.87**	0.839-0.910	3.02**	2.828-3.225
50+	1.62**	1.546-1.702	3.17**	2.985-3.370	7.41**	6.593-8.337
Education						
Some HS, no degree	1.00		1.00		1.00	
HS degree	1.30**	1.239-1.365	1.96**	1.873-2.054	0.78**	0.720-0.840
Some college	1.41**	1.344-1.481	1.45**	1.383-1.524	0.71**	0.661-0.772
BA, BS	1.58**	1.505-1.661	0.88*	0.819-0.952	1.40**	1.268-1.553
How religious are you?						
Not at all	1.00		1.00		1.00	
Not very	1.16**	1.106-1.205	0.50**	0.455-0.552	0.50**	0.442-0.555
Somewhat	1.11**	1.068-1.159	0.44**	0.406-0.482	0.61**	0.549-0.670
Very	0.97	0.915-1.017	0.51**	0.464-0.553	1.03	0.923-1.157
Religious attendance						
Never	1.00		1.00		1.00	
Less than once a month	0.84**	0.809-0.868	1.25**	1.182-1.329	0.56**	0.518-0.608
1-3 times a month	0.65**	0.615-0.677	1.24**	1.164-1.317	0.23**	0.205-0.250
About once a week	0.72**	0.679-0.755	1.08*	1.010-1.148	0.25**	0.230-0.280
More than once a week	0.58**	0.544-0.618	0.83**	0.775-0.893	0.66**	0.588-0.735
Seek comfort through religion						
Never	1.00		1.00		1.00	
Rarely	0.67**	0.641-0.705	1.91**	1.730-2.107	1.05	0.931-1.189
Sometimes	1.03	0.985-1.073	1.34**	1.240-1.446	2.32**	2.109-2.560
Often	0.96**	0.916-0.997	1.25**	1.157-1.346	2.06**	1.858-2.282
Help with daily chores						
None of the time	1.00		1.00		1.00	
A little of the time	0.64**	0.597-0.678	0.42**	0.383-0.458	0.40**	0.334-0.479
Some of the time	0.90**	0.848-0.962	0.83**	0.769-0.885	1.46**	1.299-1.632
Most of the time	0.76**	0.723-0.806	0.76**	0.707-0.811	0.75**	0.670-0.830
All of the time	0.94**	0.899-0.993	0.73**	0.677-0.775	2.34**	2.162-2.661
Someone to love						
None of the time	1.00		1.00		1.00	
A little of the time	0.46**	0.421-0.498	1.24**	1.100-1.391	1.59**	1.346-1.885
Some of the time	0.63**	0.585-0.679	1.63**	1.481-1.798	1.15	0.991-1.343
Most of the time	0.82**	0.764-0.881	1.97**	1.787-2.181	1.27*	1.091-1.482
All of the time	1.05	0.977-1.125	2.12**	1.923-2.336	1.42**	1.223-1.657

TABLE 2 (continued)

Variables	White		African American		Hispanic	
	Exp(B)	95% C.I.	Exp(B)	95% C.I.	Exp(B)	95% C.I.
Someone to give you money						
None of the time	1.00		1.00		1.00	
A little of the time	0.73**	0.689-0.768	1.25**	1.171-1.338	0.55**	0.485-0.614
Some of the time	1.03	0.981-1.090	1.03	0.970-1.099	0.64**	0.579-0.707
Most of the time	1.02	0.969-1.067	0.85**	0.792-0.907	0.61**	0.553-0.682
All of the time	0.78**	0.739-0.813	2.94**	2.767-3.129	0.58**	0.524-0.639
Constant	1.24**		0.38**		0.38**	
Nagelkerke R square		6.0		16.5		26.0

$*p < 0.005$; $**p < 0.001$

counterparts. The lowest odds (0.66) were for Hispanic females. The odds of treatment adherence increased with age in all ethnic groups, but especially for Hispanics. For example, Hispanic patients 50 and older were 7.41 times more likely than those between 18 and 34 years of age to be treatment adherent. The odds of being adherent to treatments also increased for Whites but varied for African American and Hispanic patients as educational levels increased.

While we expected a positive association between religious variables and treatment adherence, we did not find clear support for this statement. Of the three religious variables (how religious are you, religious attendance, seek comfort through religion), two had positive influences on treatment adherence for African Americans compared to just one for Whites (How religious are you?) and Hispanics (Seek comfort through religion).

For African Americans, "religious attendance" and "seek comfort through religion" positively influenced treatment adherence, with "seek comfort through religion" having the strongest influence. For example, African Americans patients who reported that they sought comfort through religion "often," "sometimes," or even "rarely" were 1.25 times, 1.34 times, and 1.91 times, respectively, more likely to be adherent to medications than African American patients who never sought comfort through religion. However, just being religious (How religious are you?) did not have any positive influence on treatment adherence. For example, African American patients who were "very" religious were only .51 times as likely to be adherent as those patients who were "not at all" religious.

For Hispanics, only "seek comfort through religion" was found to increase the likelihood of treatment adherence, but the variable had a strong effect. Hispanic patients who sought comfort through religion "sometimes" or "often" were twice as likely to be adherent as those who never turned to religion for comfort. On the other hand, significant variables for "How religious are you?" and "Religious attendance" indicate that these two measures of religiosity were not associated with any positive influence on adherence.

Finally, our findings indicate that Whites benefited from being religious (How religious are you?), though not from attending religious services or finding comfort in religion. Whites who were "not very" or "somewhat religious" were 1.16 times and 1.11 times, respectively, more likely than Whites who were "not at all religious" to be treatment adherent.

For the social support variables, having "someone to love" and "someone to give you money" were found to increase the odds that a patient was adherent, especially for Hispanics and African Americans. African American patients who had someone to love "all of the time" were 2.12 times more likely to be adherent than those who reported "none of the time." For Hispanics, the odds of being adherent were 1.42 times higher for patients who reported they had someone to love them "all of the time" compared to patients who reported "none of the time." Also, among African Americans, patients who reported they had someone to give them money "all of the time" were 2.94 times more likely to be adherent to medications compared to patients who reported "none of the time." This variable was not associated with an increased likelihood of being adherent for Whites and Hispanics.

DISCUSSION AND IMPLICATIONS

The purpose of this study was to examine the differential effects of social and religious support variables, in addition to background characteristics on treatment adherence for White, African-American, and Hispanic patients with HIV/AIDS. Bivariate analyses showed significant variations in the status of treatment adherence among these three racial and ethnic groups. That is, results showed that Whites are more likely to adhere to their antiretroviral treatment regimen, followed by African Americans and Hispanics.

Results from the multivariate analysis have some other important findings and implications. First, at the theoretical level, religious support, in addition to other types of social support, appears to be appropriate in studying treatment adherence among HIV-infected persons. Although the influence of social support on treatment adherence has been discussed in the literature, studies seldom mention the influence of religious support on treatment adherence. In this study, we assumed that HIV-infected persons seek out varieties of ways to adjust to their life-threatening disease, particularly in environments where there is social stigma. We also assumed that, similar to other types of social support from friends and families, the religious support that HIV-infected individuals receive from churchgoers and clergy as well as the comfort received through spirituality would influence treatment adherence.

Second, we found differential effects of social support, religion, and background characteristics on treatment adherence for Whites, Hispanics, and African Americans. These results suggest that strategies developed by social service providers to improve treatment adherence must be culturally appropriate. In general, the background characteristics—and some religious variables—were indicators of predicted adherence among Whites. For Whites, unlike for Hispanics and African Americans, the selected background variables, age and education, were found to be *both* statistically significant and in the expected direction, particularly in the case of the effect of the level of education on treatment adherence.

Our findings highlight the importance of social service providers working with and involving religious organizations in an effort to increase adherence and support to HIV-infected members of the African American and Hispanic communities. For African Americans and Hispanics, religion and social support, in addition to background characteristics were important determinants of treatment adherence. This finding supports that of other research showing that African Americans and Latinos are more likely than Whites to use religious/spiritually-based coping resources. For example, a recent study found that African Americans and Latinos with HIV/AIDS were more likely than Whites to turn to religious advisers for help or support (Reilly & Woo, 2004). The strong influence of religion in the African American and Latino communities is evident not only in the results of our multivariate analysis (Table 2), but also in Table 1. These findings suggest that religious or faith-based organizations in African American and Latino communities have the potential not only to provide HIV/AIDS patients with the support they need to adhere to their medication, but also to become a strong mechanism to provide HIV/AIDS education and prevention and intervention efforts. Though much has been written both about the denial of

HIV/AIDS and extreme homophobia in the African American and Latino communities, including its religious institutions, there is a paucity of research examining the attitudes of African American or Latino church members and/or clergy towards assisting persons living with HIV/AIDS (Dalton, 1989; Diaz, 1998). Further, even though this homophobia might have been a problem in the past, attitudes can change over time. More research needs to be done on this topic.

African Americans, especially, appear to have a need for financial assistance to increase their likelihood of being adherent. In fact, competing subsistence needs were found to be a barrier to receiving care for nonwhites, drug users, persons in lower socioeconomic groups (lower education and income), and the uninsured in a study conducted by Cunningham et al. (1999) using baseline data from the HCSUS dataset. Our measure of socioeconomic status–education–indicated two things: (1) both African Americans and Hispanics in our study had lower educational attainment levels than Whites; and (2) the educational attainment levels for African Americans and Hispanics were similar (Table 1). One question this raises is why the need for financial assistance was reflected for African Americans and not for Hispanics. The impact of competing subsistence needs on access to care for these two population groups is an area that needs to be further investigated.

While the analytical model seems to be appropriate in understanding treatment adherence among racial and ethnic groups, study limitations should be noted. First, limitations associated with self-reported data apply to the present study. Since the measures of treatment adherence are based on self-report, one may suspect an overestimation of these estimates. However, studies have shown that there is a positive association between treatment adherence and viral count. Other limitations are the variables used to measure social support and religious support. For example, questions measuring social support reflect only companionship and assistance. Questions measuring informational and appraisal support are not included in the survey. Similarly, religious support variables need more in depth coverage on instrumental and expressive support variables. Another major limitation of the study is the definition of treatment adherence being treated as a dichotomous variable. Although this definition is used in other studies such as Tucker et al. (2003), attention to refining this variable is indicated. Future studies might test other variations of treatment regimens and adherence/non adherence response categories. In sum, results from this study suggest the importance of additional investigation to understand the relationship of social and religious support on treatment adherence.

REFERENCES

Ajouch, K., Antonucci, T. C., & Janevic, M. R. (2001). Social networks among blacks and whites: The interaction between race and age. *Journal of Gerontology: Social Sciences, 56B,* S112-S118.

Avants, S. K., Warburton, L. A., & Margolin, A. (2001). Spiritual and religious support in recovery from addiction among HIV-positive injection drug users. *Journal of Psychoactive Drugs, 33*(1), 39-45.

Bangsberg, D. R., Perry, S., Charlebois, E., Clark, R., Robertson, M., & Moss, A. R. (2001). Adherence to HAART predicts progression to AIDS. *AIDS, 15*(9), 1181-1183.

Berkman, L. F., Glass T., Brissette, I., & Seeman, T. E. (2000). From social integration to health: Durkheim in the new millennium. *Social Science and Medicine, 51,* 843-857.

Blythe, B. J. (1983). Social support networks in health care and health promotion. In J.K. Whittaker & J. Garbarino (Eds.), *Social support networks: Informal helping in the human services* (107-127). New York: Aldine de Gruyter.

Broman, C. (1987). Race differences in professional help-seeking. *American Journal of Community Psychology, 15,* 473-489.

Catz, S. L., Kelly, J. A., Bogart, L. M., Benotsch, E. G., & McAuliffe, T. L. (2000). Patterns, correlates, and barriers to medication adherence among persons prescribed new treatments for HIV disease. *Health Psychology, 19*(2), 124-133.

Catz, S. L., McClure, J. B., Jones, G. N., & Brantley, P. J. (1999). Predictors of outpatient medical appointment attendance among persons with HIV. *AIDS Care, 11*(3), 361-373.

Centers for Disease Control and Prevention. (2002). *HIV/AIDS surveillance report 2002, 14.* Retrieved December 1, 2004 from http://www.cdc.gov/hiv/stats/hasrlink.htm.

Cohen, S., & Wills, T. A. (1985). Stress, social support, and the buffering hypothesis. *Psychological Bulletin, 98,* 310-357.

Cunningham, W. E., Andersen, R. M., Katz, M. H., Stein, M. D., Turner, B. J., Crystal, S. et al. (1999). The impact of competing subsistence needs and barriers on access to medical care for persons with Human Immunodeficiency Virus receiving care in the United States. *Medical Care, 37*(12), 1270-1281.

Dalton, H. L. (1989). AIDS in blackface. *Daedalus, 118*(3), 205-227.

Diaz, R. M. (1998). *Latino gay men and HIV: Culture, sexuality and risk behavior.* New York and London: Routledge.

Du Bois, W. E. B. (2000). *Du Bois on religion* (P. Zuckerman Ed.). New York: Alta Mira Press.

Frankel, M. R., Shapiro, M. F., Duan, N., Morton, S. C., Berry, S. H., Brown, J. A. et al. (1999). National probability samples in studies of low-prevalence diseases, part II: Designing and implementing the HIV Cost and Services Utilization Study sample. *Health Services Research, 34*(5 pt 2), 969-992.

Gant, L. M., & Ostrow, D. G. (1995). Perceptions of social support and psychological adaptation to sexually acquired HIV among White and African American men. *Social Work, 40,* 215-224.

Golin, C. E., Liu, H., Hays, R. D., Miller, L. G., Beck, C. K., Ickovics, J. et al. (2002). A prospective study of predictors of adherence to combination antiretroviral medication. *Journal of General Internal Medicine, 17,* 756-765.

Hall, B. A. (1994). Ways of maintaining hope in HIV disease. *Research in Nursing & Health, 17*, 283-293.

Heckman, T. G., Kochman, A., Sikkema, K. J., Kalichman, S. C., Masten, J., & Goodkin, K. (2000). Late middle-aged and older men living with HIV/AIDS: Race differences in coping, social support, and psychological distress. *Journal of the National Medical Association, 92*(9), 436-444.

Hill, P. C., & Pargament, K. I. (2003). Advances in the conceptualization and measurement of religion and spirituality: Implications for physical and mental health research. *American Psychologist, 58*, 64-74.

Hill, P. C., Pargament, K. I., Hood, R. W., McCullough, M. E., Swyers, J. P., Larson, D. B. et al. (2000). Conceptualizing religion and spirituality: Points of commonality, points of departure. *Journal for the Theory of Social Behavior, 30*, 51-77.

James, W. (1961). *The varieties of religious experiences: A study in human nature.* Cambridge, MA: Harvard University Press.

Jones, G. N., Catz, S. I., McClure, J. B., Jeffries, S. K., & Baglio, C. (1996). Coping patterns among low SES HIV-infected individuals [abstract]. *AABT 30th Annual Convention Proceedings.*

Krause, N. (2002). Exploring race differences in a comprehensive battery of church-based social support measures. *Review of Religious Research, 44*, 126-149.

Krause, N. (2003). Exploring race differences in the relationship between social interaction with the clergy and feelings of self-worth in late life. *Sociology of Religion, 64*(2), 183-205.

Meichenbaum, D., & Turk, D. C. (1987). *Facilitating treatment adherence: A practitioner's guidebook.* New York: Plenum Press.

Mertler, C. A., & Vannatta, R. A. (2004). *Advanced and multivariate statistical methods: Practical application and interpretation (3rd ed.).* Los Angeles, CA: Pyrczak Publishing.

Mullen, P. M., Smith, R. M., & Hill, E. W. (1993). Sense of coherence as a mediator of stress for cancer patients and spouses. *Journal of Psychosocial Oncology, 11*, 23-46.

Neighbors, H., & Jackson, J. S. (1987). Barriers to medical care among adult blacks: What happens to the uninsured? *Journal of the National Medical Association, 79*, 489-493.

Palella, F. J., Jr., Delaney, K. M., Moorman, A. C., Loveless, M. O., Fuhrer, J., Satten, G. A. et al. (1998). Declining morbidity and mortality among patients with advanced human immunodeficiency virus infection. *New England Journal of Medicine, 338*(13), 853-860.

Pargament, K. I. (1997). *The psychology of religion and coping: Theory, research, practice.* New York: Guilford Press.

Pargament, K. I. (1990). God help me: Toward a theoretical framework of coping for the psychology of religion. *Research in the social scientific study of religion, 2*, 195-224.

Pargament, K. I., & Hahn, J. (1986). God and the just world: Causal and coping attributions to God in health situations. *Journal for the Scientific Study of Religion, 25*, 193-207.

Paterson, D. L., Swindells, S., Mohr, J., Brester, M., Vergis, E. N., Squier, C. et al. (2000). Adherence to protease inhibitor therapy and outcomes in patients with HIV infection. *Annals of Internal Medicine, 133*(1), 21-30.

Power, R., Koopman, C., Volk, J., Israelski, D. M., Stone, L., Chesney, M. A. et al. (2003). Social support, substance use, and denial in relationship to antiretroviral treatment adherence among HIV-infected persons. *AIDS Patient Care and STDs, 17*(5), 245-252.

Reilly, T., & Woo, G. (2004). Social support and maintenance of safer sex practices among people living with HIV/AIDS. *Health and Social Work, 29*(2), 97-105.

Rogers, R. G. (1996). The effects of family composition, health, and social support linkages on mortality. *Journal of Health and Social Behavior, 37*(4), 326-338.

Rogers, R. G., Hummer, R. A., & Nam, C. B. (2000). *Living and dying in the USA.* San Diego, CA: Academic Press.

Schwarzer, F., Dunkel-Schetter, C., & Kemeny, M. (1994). The multidimensional nature of received social support in gay men at risk of HIV infection and AIDS. *American Journal of Community Psychology, 22*(3), 319-339.

Shapiro, M. F., Berk, M. L., Berry, S. H., Emmons, C., Athey, L. A., Hsia, D. C. et al. (1999). National probability samples in studies of low-prevalence diseases, part I: Perspectives and lessons from the HIV Cost and Services Utilization Study. *Health Services Research, 34*(5 pt 1), 951-968.

Shapiro, M. F., Morton, S. C., McCaffrey, D. F., Senterfitt, J. W., Fleishman, J. A., Perlman, J. F. et al. (1999). Variations in the care of HIV-infected adults in the United States: Results from the HIV Cost and Services Utilization Study. *Journal of American Medical Association, 281*(24), 2305-2315.

Siegel, K., & Raveis, V. (1997). Perceptions of access to HIV-related information, care, and services among infected minority men. *Qualitative Health Research, 7*(1), 9-31.

Simoni, J. M., Martone, M. G., & Kerwin, J. F. (2002). Spirituality and psychological adaptation among women with HIV/AIDS: Implications for counseling. *Journal of Counseling Psychology, 49*(2), 39-147.

Snowden, L. R. (1998). Racial differences in informal help seeking for mental health problems. *Journal of Community Psychology, 26*, 429-438.

Tucker, J. S., Burnam, M. A., Sherbourne, C. D., Kung, F. Y., & Glifford, A. L. (2003). Substance use and mental health correlates of nonadherence to antiretroviral medications in a sample of patients with human immunodeficiency virus infection. *American Journal of Medicine, 114*(7), 573-580.

Williams, A., & Friedland, G. (1997). Adherence, compliance, and HAART. *AIDS Clinical Care, 9*(7), 51-55.

Williams, D. R., Larson, D. V., Buckler, R. E., Heckman, R. C., & Pyle, C. M. (1991). Religion and psychological distress in a community sample. *Social Science and Medicine, 32*(11), 1257-1262.

Wright, M. T. (2000). The old problem of adherence: Research on treatment adherence and its relevance for HIV/AIDS. *AIDS Care, 12*(6), 703-710.

Wuthnow, R. (1998). *After heaven: Spirituality in America since the 1950s.* Berkeley: University of California Press.

Zuckerman, D. M., Kasl, S. V., & Ostfeld, A. M. (1984). Psychosocial predictors of mortality among the elderly poor: The role of religion, well-being, and social contacts. *American Journal of Epidemiology, 119*(3), 410-423.

doi:10.1300/J187v06n01_06

The Development and Feasibility of an Intervention to Improve HAART Adherence Among HIV-Positive Patients Receiving Primary Care in Methadone Clinics

Nina A. Cooperman, PsyD
Jeffrey T. Parsons, PhD
Brenda Chabon, PhD
Karina M. Berg, MD
Julia H. Arnsten, MD

SUMMARY. We developed an adherence counseling program to help HIV-positive, opioid dependent patients, receiving primary care in methadone clinics, to improve adherence to highly active antiretroviral therapy (HAART). The intervention is conducted by paraprofessional

---

Nina A. Cooperman, PsyD, Brenda Chabon, PhD, and Karina M. Berg, MD, are all Assistant Professors; and Julia H. Arnsten, MD, is Associate Professor and Chief of the Division of General Internal Medicine; all affiliated with Albert Einstein College of Medicine and Montefiore Medical Center, Bronx, NY.

Jeffrey T. Parsons, PhD, is Professor, Hunter College and the Graduate Center of the City University of New York, and the Director of the Center for HIV/AIDS Educational Studies and Training.

Address correspondence to: Nina A. Cooperman, Montefiore Medical Center, Division of General Internal Medicine, 111 East 210th Street, Bronx, NY 10467 (E-mail: nicooperm@montefiore.org).

[Haworth co-indexing entry note]: "The Development and Feasibility of an Intervention to Improve HAART Adherence Among HIV-Positive Patients Receiving Primary Care in Methadone Clinics." Cooperman, Nina A. et al. Co-published simultaneously in *the Journal of HIV/AIDS & Social Services* (The Haworth Press, Inc.) Vol. 6, No. 1/2, 2007, pp. 101-120; and: *HIV Treatment Adherence: Challenges for Social Services* (ed: Lana Sue Ka'opua and Nathan L. Linsk) The Haworth Press, Inc., 2007, pp. 101-120. Single or multiple copies of this article are available for a fee from The Haworth Document Delivery Service [1-800-HAWORTH, 9:00 a.m. - 5:00 p.m. (EST). E-mail address: docdelivery@haworthpress.com].

adherence counselors and consists of six, semi-structured counseling sessions that focus on motivational interviewing and cognitive-behavioral skills training. To date, we have enrolled 119 patients into adherence counseling, suggesting that patients are interested and receptive to the program. Clinic staff has welcomed the additional support provided by the program, and are working collaboratively with the adherence counselors to provide integrated and comprehensive care. The successful implementation of the adherence counseling program indicates that paraprofessionals can effectively be trained to provide semi-structured adherence counseling and that adherence interventions can be incorporated into existing substance abuse and HIV-related treatment programs.

doi:10.1300/J187v06n01_07 *[Article copies available for a fee from The Haworth Document Delivery Service: 1-800-HAWORTH. E-mail address: <docdelivery@haworthpress.com> Website: <http://www.HaworthPress.com>*

KEYWORDS. Adherence, compliance, HIV, AIDS, HAART, intervention, counseling, antiretroviral medication

INTRODUCTION

With the development of highly active antiretroviral therapy (HAART), HIV-positive individuals now have the opportunity to live prolonged, active, and productive lives. However, adherence to the often complex HAART regimens must be almost perfect (over 95%) for the medications to be effective (Patterson et al., 2000). In New York City, approximately 40% of those with HIV were infected through injection drug use and factors that may adversely affect adherence (poverty, addiction, depression, and poor education) are highly prevalent among substance users (Arnsten et al., 2002; Carballo et al., 2004; NYC Department of Health, 2003; Reynolds et al., 2004; Sharpe, Lee, Elam-Evans, & Fleming, 2004; Tucker, Burnam, Sherbourne, & Kung, 2003). While the opportunity to prevent the advancement of HIV and AIDS exists, many individuals with substance abuse problems do not receive the same benefit from HAART as compared to other groups. Drug treatment programs have attempted to address the burden of HIV/AIDS through testing programs, risk education, service referral, and medical care; however, physicians, substance abuse counselors, and social workers in substance abuse treatment settings often lack the time, training, experience, and resources to effectively address medication adherence among HIV-positive individuals.

We developed the Support for Treatment Adherence Readiness (STAR) Program, an intervention combining motivational interviewing and cognitive-behavioral techniques, to improve HAART adherence among HIV-positive substance abusers receiving primary care at 12 methadone maintenance clinics in Bronx, New York. The 12 clinics are part of the Division of Substance Abuse at the Albert Einstein College of Medicine and Montefiore Medical Center, and use a treatment paradigm that relies on integrating general and HIV-related medical, substance abuse, and mental health services under one roof. Our adherence program exemplifies the incorporation of an innovative HIV-related treatment service into existing methadone treatment programs. Four paraprofessionals were trained in motivational interviewing and the provision of a semi-structured adherence counseling program. We sought to determine feasibility of this program by evaluating patient interest and enrollment, acceptance and cooperation by clinic staff, and ability of the paraprofessional counselors to learn and implement motivational interviewing and the semi-structured adherence counseling program. The successful implementation of this program in a system that provides primary care to over 500 HIV-positive individuals indicates that paraprofessionals can be effectively trained to supplement the services of medical, social work, mental health, and substance abuse professionals in the care of the HIV-infected patients in methadone maintenance.

LITERATURE REVIEW

Barriers to Adherence

While almost perfect adherence is required for HAART to be effective and to prevent resistance, studies have shown that in the general medical population, 50% of patients are non-adherent to their prescribed medication regimens (Sorensen et al., 1998; Wright, 2000). Lack of adherence in general is so common that no grouping of sociodemographic characteristics can reliably predict it (Wright). Nonetheless, particular emphasis has been given to defining correlates of adherence among drug users for several reasons: drug users account for an increasing proportion of prevalent AIDS cases in many urban centers, drug users are traditionally thought to be less capable of adhering to medical treatments, and there is concern that poor adherence among persons engaging in high risk behaviors will foster the development and transmission of resistant virus strains (Bogart, Kelly, Catz, & Sosman, 2000; Catz, Kelly, Bogart, Benotsch, & McAuliffe, 2000; Holmberg, 1996; Salomon et al., 2000). In fact, active drug or alcohol abuse has been found to be one of a few relatively consistent predictors of poor adherence across studies (Arnsten et al., 2002; Ferrando, Wall, Batki, & Sorensen, 1996; Haubrich, Little, Currier, Forthal, & Kemper, 1999; Lucas, Cheever, Chaisson, & Moore, 2001). However, past history of drug or alcohol abuse has not been consistently associated with poor adherence, and a number of studies have found that persons not actively using drugs, as well as some active users, are able to adhere to antiretroviral treatments with success comparable to that of non-drug users (Arnsten et al., 2001; Holzemer et al., 1999; Lucas et al., 2001).

For both active and former drug users, engagement in substance abuse treatment, particularly if on-site primary care is available, appears to facilitate access and adherence to HAART and other medical therapies (Celentano et al., 1998; Samet, Friedmann, & Saitz, 2001; Selwyn, Budner, Wasserman, & Arno, 1997). Among both drug users and non drug users, social stability and support, beliefs and knowledge about medications, and confidence in the ability to take HIV medications (including both self-efficacy and "fit" with daily activities) have consistently been identified as predictors of adherence (Catz et al., 2000; Gao, Nau, Rosenbluth, Scott, & Woodward, 2000; Kalichman, Ramachandran, & Catz, 1999; Safren et al., 2000). In addition, active mental illness, particularly depression, has been associated with poor adherence in many studies (Avants, Margolin, Warburton, Hawkins, & Shi, 2001; Catz et al.; Holzemer et al., 1999; Safren et al.). Some other common reasons for non-adherence have also been reported across studies, and include difficulty remembering, inconvenient dosing, and medication side effects (Catz et al.; Ostrop, Hallett, & Gill, 2000).

Adherence Intervention Research

Emerging research has shown that some short-term interventions focusing on adherence to antiretroviral medications may improve adherence and related health outcomes. McPherson-Baker et al. (2000) found that 21 HIV-positive men who received five monthly individual medication counseling sessions and were provided with a weekly medication organizer had greater medication adherence and clinic visits, and fewer hospitalizations and opportunistic infections as compared to matched controls who received standard care. Among 23 HIV-positive adolescents and young adults, aged 15-22 years, Lyon et al. (2003) evaluated an adherence intervention that included six biweekly family and youth education sessions. The participants were given pillboxes, calendars, and watch alarms. The researchers found that 91% of those participating in the intervention reported increased HAART adherence, as well as an increase in other health-promoting behaviors such as attendance at medical appointments, immunizations, and referrals to mental health and substance abuse treatment. Tuldra et al. (2000) reported that 55 HIV-positive men and women who received a psychoeducational intervention based on Bandura's self-efficacy theory had greater adherence and were more likely to have an undetectable viral load than 61 similar individuals who received routine medical care.

In contrast, other studies have described interventions that are ineffective or provide only temporary results. Rigsby et al. (2000) provided cue-dose training (i.e., training to help subjects identify cues to help them remember to take their medications) to one group of HIV-positive subjects, cue-dose training with a monetary incentive to a second group of subjects, and non-directive inquiries about adherence to a control group of subjects. Compared to the control group, the researchers did not find significant increases in adherence among those who received cue-dose training alone or non-directive inquiries. They did find greater adherence among the subjects who received cue dose training and cash reinforcement as compared to the control group only; however, the increase in adherence was not maintained long-term. In another study, HIV-positive individuals randomized into a treatment focusing on empowerment and medication adherence skill building were compared to a similar group of individuals who received only basic education about taking their medications (Rawlings et al., 2003). In this study, adherence in the treatment group did not improve compared to the control group.

Simoni, Frick, Pantalone, and Turner (2003) conducted a review of the literature on antiretroviral adherence interventions. The review included 21 published studies which evaluated cognitive, behavioral, and affective adherence interventions, and abstracts of ongoing National Institutes of Health funded projects. Overall, while a few studies did not show improved adherence after the administration of an adherence intervention, the majority reported that counseling or support had a significant positive impact on medication adherence. The authors concluded that current research suggests that strategies such as assessing and helping patients cope with barriers to adherence, providing social support, and implementing cognitive and behavioral techniques to improve medication adherence are effective.

Parsons, Rosof, Punzalan, and DiMaria (2005) recently piloted an intervention designed to improve medication adherence and decrease substance use among HIV-positive substance abusers in New York City. The intervention, which helped to inform the STAR Program, demonstrated feasibility and acceptability, and had a significant impact on reducing substance use and a trend towards an impact on improving medication adherence. Delivered by highly trained therapists over eight sessions, it is unclear how such counseling interventions can be delivered by a broader range of health care providers.

Adherence Counseling Practice

While counseling to improve adherence to HAART is warranted and some interventions have been shown to be effective for improving adherence, the training and skill of healthcare providers varies widely and the implementation of adherence counseling programs is inconsistent (Golin, Smith, & Reif, 2004; Reif, Smith, & Golin, 2003; Roberts & Voldberding, 1999). In fact, a study investigating the practices of 94 HIV/AIDS case managers in the southern United States reported that while the majority of the case managers discussed medications with their patients, many felt that their adherence counseling skills were inadequate (Reif et al., 2003). In addition, significant variability in adherence counseling interventions was found, with most counselors providing medication monitoring and fewer providing medication education, instructions, or counseling.

Although most physicians agree that adherence counseling is important for HIV-positive patients on HAART, the degree and quality of the counseling provided by physicians varies. Among physicians who treat HIV-positive patients in North Carolina, almost all (97%) reported that they view adherence counseling as important and part of their role; however, nearly 50% reported that they do not have enough time to provide the counseling. The physicians spent, on average, 13 minutes counseling patients beginning a new antiretroviral regimen, and 7.5 min during follow-up visits. Most of the physicians reported giving basic dosing instructions, but a minority provided counseling on remembering medications, planning dose times, side effect management, drug interactions, or what to do if a dose is missed (Golin et al., 2004).

A qualitative study investigating provider-patient communications about adherence to HAART found that among fifteen physicians at San

Francisco General Hospital, most provided pre-prescription assessment and counseling for their HIV-positive patients, including education about the medication or how to deal with psychosocial stressors (Roberts & Volberding, 1999). On the other hand, follow-up after beginning medications generally consisted of a "checking in" on how patients were doing on their medications, and the questions about medication ranged from broad to specific. Two physicians did not provide any adherence counseling or do routine follow-ups with patients after beginning medications. These physicians relied on viral load tests as an assessment of adherence and had brief discussions about medication adherence or provided written materials for the patients to read as opposed to providing face-to-face counseling. In sum, while physicians realize the importance of adherence support and generally take time to educate their patients about adherence, they are not able to give the in depth support that many patients require. Therefore, adherence support by well-trained ancillary health providers would be extremely beneficial for both the patients and treatment teams that do not have the resources required to provide needed adherence interventions.

STAR PROGRAM

Goals

The goal of the STAR Program is to improve adherence with HAART among HIV-infected current and former opioid users enrolled in a methadone maintenance program at which on-site HIV primary care is provided. The STAR Program was designed to be comprehensive, flexible, and integrated into usual clinical care for drug users. Therefore, all HAART-eligible patients, whether or not they are currently taking HAART, are offered participation. In addition, STAR Program services are fully incorporated into both medical and drug abuse treatment, so that both medical and non-medical clinicians will be part of the adherence treatment team. The specific objectives of the STAR Program are:

1. To provide individualized adherence readiness training to patients prior to beginning or re-starting HAART.
2. To assess and monitor self-reported medication adherence, barriers to adherence, and adherence self-efficacy among patients who are currently taking HAART.

3. To provide individualized and ongoing adherence support to all patients currently taking HAART.
4. To increase the proportion of patients achieving and maintaining an undetectable viral load.

This paper reports on the feasibility of the STAR program and provides preliminary descriptive data on enrollees at baseline.

Theoretical Framework

The STAR Program is based on the Information-Motivation-Behavior Skills (IMB) model of behavior change (Fisher, Fisher, Bryan, & Misovich, 2002; Fisher, Fisher, Misovich, Kimble, & Malloy, 1996; Fisher, Fisher, Williams, & Malloy, 1994). This model asserts that information is necessary but insufficient to alter behavior and that motivation and behavioral skills are critical determinants in promoting behavior change. While information and motivation work largely through behavioral skills to affect behavior, both information and motivation can directly influence behavior as well. IMB-inspired interventions have demonstrated effectiveness in changing behavior across a variety of clinical applications, and the model has increasingly been applied to the development of interventions to improve adherence with HAART.

To enhance motivation for adherence, our intervention incorporates brief motivational interviewing (MI), a technique that was originally developed to treat substance abuse and has been shown to be successful with other health behavior change, including, but only recently, medication adherence among HIV-positive adults (Adamian, Golin, Shain, & DeVellis, 2004; Konkle-Parker, 2001; Parsons et al., 2005). The foundation of MI is the Transtheoretical Model, which proposes that behavior change is cyclical through a series of five stages: pre-contemplation, contemplation, preparation, action, and maintenance (Miller & Rollnick, 2002; Prochaska & DiClemente, 1992). According to the Transtheoretical Model, individuals may relapse and often cycle through these stages several times before making a long-lasting or permanent behavior change. MI is a non-confrontational, patient centered approach where four basic principles are utilized to amplify a patient's ambivalence about a health related behavior and support the patient through the stages of change. The four basic principles are: (1) express empathy (2) develop discrepancy (3) do not challenge resistance and (4) support self-efficacy. The spirit and philosophy of MI is one of collaboration, evocation, and autonomy, where the patient's goals and readiness to change dictate the direction of the intervention.

In addition, cognitive-behavioral skills training (CBST) is used to promote the skills necessary to create behavioral change. Overall, CBST interventions are designed to modify critical cognitions and actions that maintain problem behaviors (in this case, non-adherence to HIV medications). Some of these interventions are based on the conceptual framework of Social Cognitive Theory, which posits that behavior is determined by three factors: outcome expectancies, self-efficacy, and coping skills (Bandura, 1986). CBST interventions help a person identify operative antecedents of a behavior and subsequently teach skills to cope with the proximal risk antecedents for that behavior. It has been suggested that many CBST interventions could be improved by having the skills training component be guided by a functional analysis of an individual patient, rather than teaching a narrow set of skills and delivering them in a uniform manner (Morgenstern, Kahler, & Epstein, 1998). For this reason, a functional analysis of missed medication is conducted as a part of the STAR Program, and counselors work with patients to develop individualized goals.

Program Structure

Our semi-structured adherence intervention consists of six (30-40 minute) sessions, incorporating motivational interviewing and cognitive-behavioral techniques, modified from the pilot intervention of Parsons et al. (2005) (see Table 1). The first two sessions are MI-driven, semi-structured, and focus on assessing adherence obstacles, determining stage of change, eliciting change talk, determining triggers for non-adherence, and developing treatment goals. The following four sessions are more cognitive-behavioral, and focus on HIV adherence education and skill development, tailored to the patient's needs and goals. Structured modules such as developing a social network, communicating with providers, memory strategies, self-care, increasing pleasant activities, coping with side effects, and challenging distorted thoughts are implemented to facilitate skill building. Patients are also educated about treatment resistance, risk behavior, and myths about HIV and antiretroviral medications. The adherence counselors work to identify unaddressed mental health, substance abuse, financial, vocational, and housing issues that are potentially impeding HIV medication adherence, and collaborate with the treatment team (physician, physician assistant, social worker, and substance abuse counselor) to provide appropriate

TABLE 1. STAR Program Structure and Content

Session	Theme	Activities
Session 1	Assessment	Establish rapport, structured and unstructured assessment. Incorporate motivational interviewing techniques. Identify stage of change and triggers for non-adherence. Make referrals as needed.[a]
Session 2	Goal setting	Assessment of adherence. Goal setting and development of change plan. Incorporate motivational interviewing techniques. Make referrals as needed.
Session 3	Education and skill building	Assessment of adherence. Provide and review educational materials.[b] Provide and review skill building modules.[c] Make referrals as needed.
Session 4	Education and skill building	Assessment of adherence. Provide and review educational materials. Provide and review skill building modules. Make referrals as needed.
Session 5	Education and skill building	Assessment of adherence. Provide and review educational materials. Provide and review skill building modules. Make referrals as needed.
Session 6	Relapse prevention	Evaluate progress since first session. Summarize previous sessions and validate effort/changes made. Discuss relapse triggers and prevention. Talk about future "booster sessions" and other avenues for support. Make referrals as needed.
"Booster" sessions	As needed[d]	Assessment. May provide relapse prevention, develop new goals and change plan, provide and review educational materials and modules. Make referrals as needed.

[a] Work with substance abuse counselor, social worker, physician, or physician assistant to obtain additional mental health or social services.

[b] For example, what HIV is and how the virus impacts the immune system, how antiretroviral medications work, resistance, myths and facts, when and how to take specific regimens.

[c] For example, coping with triggers, communication with providers, managing thoughts, managing side effects, making time for yourself, increasing social support, increasing pleasant activities.

[d] Participant may begin medications at a later date, begin a new regimen, enter a new stage of change, encounter new stressors, health may change etc. If necessary, participant may receive an additional six sessions at a later date.

intervention and referrals. The final session focuses on relapse prevention and identifying future goals. After treatment termination, patients are provided with "booster sessions," as needed, and are eligible to enter the full treatment again if their circumstances change (for example, a new medication regimen, change in life circumstances, or transition to a different stage of change).

Assessment

During the first STAR Program visit, adherence counselors, using a structured questionnaire, ask patients about demographic information, and possible mode of HIV transmission. They also collect baseline information regarding current CD4 count, viral load, psychiatric diagnoses, symptoms of depression, substance use, and whether they are prescribed antiretroviral medication. If the patient is prescribed medication, the counselor asks for the names of the medications, how often the patient misses doses, and methods used to remember to take the medications. At the first visit, to further clarify adherence obstacles, the counselor may ask additional unstructured questions about social support, knowledge about HIV and antiretroviral medication, physical health, disclosure, and relationships with providers. During each subsequent session, the adherence counselor fills out, with the patient, a brief questionnaire that asks whether the patient is on antiretrovirals, and if yes, adherence during the past month, week, and three days. For as long as the participants are willing to be reassessed, information collected at baseline and with the questionnaires at counseling visits is again collected from STAR Program participants at follow-up assessments every three months, regardless of the number of adherence counseling sessions attended. This information is used to determine the necessity of booster sessions or re-entering the full counseling program. Data was abstracted from patient charts and de-identified for the descriptive analyses described in this paper.

Training

Prior to the implementation of the STAR Program in our substance abuse treatment program, the purpose and logistics of the program were explained to all clinic administrators, counselors, social workers, and primary care providers at divisional and clinic staff meetings. The adherence counselors, clinic physicians, physician assistants, and HIV care coordinators were then provided with a two-day training on motivational interviewing, delivered by an experienced MI trainer and co-developer of the intervention. The adherence counselors received additional HIV-specific training from an infectious disease physician and training by a clinical psychologist on the specifics of the counseling structure and the psychosocial issues that could impact medication adherence. Since the STAR Program has been implemented, the adherence counselors have been receiving ongoing training and supervision by our staff clinical psychologist and our MI trainer. The counselors meet with the psychologist for weekly group and individual supervision. During the supervision, audiotapes of the counseling sessions are reviewed, and further in-depth training on issues related to HIV and the counseling is conducted (e.g., risk behavior, partner notification, referral resources, ethics, relaxation techniques, suicide assessment). The counselors are encouraged to share their knowledge and resources with other clinic staff. We abstracted data from patient charts which were de-identified for the descriptive analysis.

RESULTS

Preliminary Findings

To date, 119 patients have enrolled in the STAR Program (Table 2), 18 have completed all 6 sessions, and 18 have withdrawn from the program. Of the 18 patients who have withdrawn from the program, 5 refused services, 11 felt they didn't need services, 1 was incarcerated, and 1 died. The majority of those enrolled is female (59%), Hispanic (57%), and live in a house or apartment that they rent or own (72%). Almost all patients (95%) received their HIV diagnosis more than three years ago, with injection drug use (38%) as the most commonly reported HIV-risk behavior. Over half of the patients (54%) self-reported having a diagnosis of depression, and half reported feeling depressed during the week prior to their first session. During the month prior to their first session, almost a quarter of the patients used cocaine or crack.

While 67% percent were currently prescribed antiretroviral medication at the time of their first counseling session, only 32% of patients enrolled in the adherence counseling had an undetectable viral load baseline. Of those prescribed antiretrovirals ($n = 57$), 27% were on their first HAART regimen. Before beginning the adherence counseling, the patients used pillboxes (43%), alarms (19%), written instructions (2%), and other means (21%) to help them remember to take their medications. On average, the patients self-reported taking their medications "most of the time" (4 on a scale that ranged from 1[never] to 5 [all of the time] and were "pretty sure" (2 on a scale that ranged from 1 [not sure] to 3 [very sure]) that their HIV medications are helping to fight the HIV virus.

TABLE 2. Descriptive Data

N = 93	%
Gender	
Male	40
Female	59
Transgender	1
Race	
Hispanic	57
Black	29
White	13
Asian/Pacific Islander	1
Housing	
Rent or own house/apartment	72
Someone else's house/apartment	14
Transitional/temporary housing	7
Hotel, HIV/AIDS housing, shelter	7
Time since diagnosis	
More than 3 years	96
1-3 years	4
Exposure to HIV	
Men sex with men	1
Injection drug use	38
Sex with an injection drug user	18
Sex with non-injection drug user	22
Blood transfusion	1
Psychiatric diagnosis (Self Report)	
Depression	54
Anxiety	12
Personality disorder	1
No diagnosis	31
Other	3
Unknown	6
Felt depressed in past week	49
Drug use during past month	
Cocaine	27
Crack	21
Heroin	15
Street or club drugs (ecstasy, special k, crystal meth)	2
Prescription pain pills or benzodiazepines	9
Regular alcohol use (3 or more drinks a day)	16
Undetectable viral load	32
CD4 (Median)	293
Viral load (Median)	8032
Prescribed antiretroviral medication	67

TABLE 2 (continued)

$n = 57^a$	%
First HAART regimen	27
Methods to remember medications	
Pillbox	43
Alarm	19
Written instructions	2
Other	21
How often medications taken during the last month (Mean)	4[b]
How sure medications will help fight HIV (Mean)	2[c]

[a] Those prescribed antiretroviral medication at first session.
[b] Patients were asked, "How often would you say you've taken your HIV medications in the past month?" and report, 1(never), 2(sometimes), 3(about half the time), 4(most of the time), or 5(all of the time).
[c] Patients were asked "How sure are you that the HIV medications you are taking will help you fight the virus?" and report 1(not sure), 2(pretty sure), or 3(very sure).

DISCUSSION

While the evaluation of the STAR Program is ongoing, and the data presented is preliminary and from baseline only, several conclusions may be drawn. First, there is a clear need for adherence counseling in methadone clinics at which on-site HIV primary care is provided. While 67% of the patients enrolled in the STAR Program had been prescribed HAART, only 32% of the patients enrolled in the STAR Program had reached undetectable viral loads. Second, patients and staff are receptive and interested in participating in adherence counseling. Within four months, 119 patients have voluntarily enrolled in adherence counseling, and additional patients will begin counseling once those initially enrolled complete the program. In addition, the substance abuse counselors, physician assistants, physicians, social workers, and other clinic administrative staff have welcomed the additional support provided by the STAR Program, and are working collaboratively with the adherence counselors to provide integrated and comprehensive care. Third, paraprofessionals can effectively be trained to provide semi-structured adherence counseling. Unlike the Parsons et al. (2005) pilot intervention which used highly trained therapists, all of our counselors had little prior experience in motivational interviewing or cognitive-behavioral skills training, and have been able to grasp and successfully apply both techniques within the structure of the six session STAR Program. As such, this intervention approach can be delivered by a broad range of providers, with varying levels of background and experience in approaches to counseling.

However, while adherence counseling seems to be both needed and feasible in the methadone maintenance treatment program setting, barriers to implementation and effectiveness exist. For example, many of the obstacles that impede adherence to HAART (substance abuse, depression, poor social support, and other psychosocial stressors) are the same as the obstacles that prevent attendance at adherence counseling appointments. Therefore, the individuals most in need for adherence counseling are the least likely to receive its benefits. We attempt to remedy this by identifying and acknowledging barriers to treatment attendance early in the counseling (often at the first session), and working with the patients to enhance motivation and develop strategies that will improve retention and adherence to the counseling structure as well as to HAART.

Given that the methadone clinic is a crowded and active environment, another issue is confidentiality. Many of the HIV-positive patients have not disclosed their status and are concerned about others identifying them as HIV-positive. Clinic patients could potentially identify HIV-positive patients by seeing who meets with the "adherence counselor." Therefore, in the clinics, we refer to the adherence counselors as simply "counselors" to prevent labeling of patients that participate in the STAR Program. However, while we attempt to maintain confidentiality, the clinics serve both HIV-positive and HIV-negative individuals, and some patients may choose not to participate because they fear being associated with a program and a counselor that focuses on HIV-specific issues.

Another difficulty in implementing the STAR Program is that the philosophy and style of the intervention differs from the often punitive climate in methadone clinics, and requires patients to adjust to the patient centered approach. In addition, the motivational interviewing foundation of the adherence intervention sometimes contrasts with the more confrontational style of some substance abuse counselors and physicians. However, through ongoing discussion with clinic staff and education about the Transtheoretical Model and techniques of motivational interviewing, we have been able to create a collaborative treatment team.

Despite these difficulties, adherence counseling in methadone clinics not only has positive implications for the health of HIV-positive, methadone maintained patients, it may also have long-term financial benefits. Non-adherent HIV-positive patients are more likely to be hospitalized and require a greater amount of medical care (Valenti, 2001). Hospitalization and increased use of medical care will likely have a greater cost than effective adherence counseling, which enables HIV-positive patients to achieve optimal adherence and receive all of the benefits of HAART, including health maintenance and the ability to remain independent and productive. Goldie et al. (2003) conducted a study evaluating the cost-effectiveness of adherence interventions (i.e., directly observed therapy, medication dispensers, beepers, alarms, and reminders) for individuals with HIV, and found that even very expensive and moderately successful adherence interventions are likely to have favorable cost-effectiveness ratios compared to no intervention, especially in an urban population such as the one served by the STAR Program.

While the STAR Program had been successfully implemented in 12 methadone maintenance clinics in the Bronx, further research is required to determine its feasibility in other settings and with other populations. In addition, analysis of follow-up data is necessary to determine whether the STAR Program helps to significantly improve patients' medication adherence, physical health and quality of life. A randomized controlled trial comparing the semi-structured counseling of the STAR Program to a control group or alternative intervention will also help to further clarify the feasibility and impact of the STAR Program on antiretroviral medication adherence.

The development and successful implementation of the STAR Program suggests a model that can be used in other substance abuse treatment programs that provide primary care for HIV-positive patients. Paraprofessionals can conduct structured adherence counseling, or professionals such as HIV-testing counselors, substance abuse counselors, or social workers can easily be trained to implement a brief adherence intervention such as the STAR Program. Moreover, adherence interventions can be incorporated into existing substance abuse and HIV-related treatment programs. With an understanding of motivational interviewing and the use of structured intervention and educational materials, those caring for HIV-positive patients in substance abuse settings can feel empowered to provide the services that they know their patients need.

ACKNOWLEDGMENTS

This work was supported by the New York State Department of Health AIDS Institute (13-1624225) and the National Institute on Drug Abuse (R01DA015302).

The authors would like to thank those who helped to develop and implement the STAR Program, Terri Febbrarro, Wendy Brown, and Daniel Kaswan, and the adherence counselors, Mark Flores, Marc King, Lisa Mosley, and Rosa Rodriguez. The authors would also like to acknowledge Denise Hernandez and Megha Ramaswamy, who helped with this manuscript.

REFERENCES

Adamian, M. S., Golin, C. E., Shain, L. S., & DeVellis, B. (2004). Brief motivational interviewing to improve adherence to antiretroviral therapy: development and qualitative pilot assessment of an intervention. *AIDS Patient Care and STDS, 18,* 229-238.

Arnsten, J. H., Demas, P. A., Farzadegan, H., Grant, R. W., Gourevitch, M. N., Chang, C. J. et al. (2001). Antiretroviral therapy adherence and viral suppression in HIV-infected drug users: comparison of self-report and electronic monitoring. *Clinical Infectious Diseases, 33,* 1417-1423.

Arnsten, J. H., Demas, P. A., Grant, R. W., Gourevitch, M. N., Farzadegan, H., Howard, A. A. et al. (2002). Impact of active drug use on antiretroviral therapy adherence and viral suppression in HIV-infected drug users. *Journal of General Internal Medicine, 17,* 377-381.

Avants, S. K., Margolin, A., Warburton, L. A., Hawkins, K. A., & Shi, H. (2001). Predictors of nonadherence to HIV-related medication regimens during methadone stabilization. *American Journal on Addictions, 10,* 69-78.

Bandura, A. (1986). *Social foundations of thought and action: A social cognitive theory.* (1 ed.) Englewood Cliffs, NJ: Prentice-Hall.

Bogart, L. M., Kelly, J. A., Catz, S. L., & Sosman, J. M. (2000). Impact of medical and nonmedical factors on physician decision making for HIV/AIDS antiretroviral treatment. *Journal of Acquired Immune Deficiency Syndromes, 23,* 396-404.

Carballo, E., Cadarso-Suarez, C. C. I., Fraga, J., Ocampo, A., Ojea, R., & Prieto, A. (2004). Assessing relationships between health-related quality of life and adherence to antiretroviral therapy. *Quality of Life Research, 13,* 587-599.

Catz, S. L., Kelly, J. A., Bogart, L. M., Benotsch, E. G., & McAuliffe, T. L. (2000). Patterns, correlates, and barriers to medication adherence among persons prescribed new treatments for HIV disease. *Health Psychology, 19,* 124-133.

Celentano, D. D., Vlahov, D., Cohn, S., Shadle, V. M., Obasanjo, O., & Moore, R. D. (1998). Self-Reported Antiretroviral Therapy in Injection Drug Users. *JAMA: The Journal of the American Medical Association, 280,* 544-546.

Ferrando, S. J., Wall, T. L., Batki, S. L., & Sorensen, J. L. (1996). Psychiatric morbidity, illicit drug use and adherence to zidovudine (AZT) among injection drug users with HIV disease. *American Journal of Drug and Alcohol Abuse, 22,* 475-487.

Fisher, J. D., Fisher, W. A., Bryan, A. D., & Misovich, S. J. (2002). Information-motivation-behavioral skills model-based HIV risk behavior change intervention for inner-city high school youth. *Health Psychology, 21,* 177-186.

Fisher, J. D., Fisher, W. A., Misovich, S. J., Kimble, D. L., & Malloy, T. E. (1996). Changing AIDS risk behavior: effects of an intervention emphasizing AIDS risk reduction information, motivation, and behavioral skills in a college student population. *Health Psychology, 15,* 114-123.

Fisher, J. D. F., Fisher, W. A. F., Williams, S. S. F., & Malloy, T. E. (1994). Empirical tests of an information-motivation-behavioral skills model of AIDS-preventive behavior with gay men and heterosexual university students. *Health Psychology, 13,* 238-250.

Gao, X., Nau, D. P., Rosenbluth, S. A., Scott, V., & Woodward, C. (2000). The relationship of disease severity, health beliefs and medication adherence among HIV patients. *AIDS Care, 12*, 387-398.

Golin, C. E., Smith, S. R., & Reif, S. (2004). Adherence counseling practices of generalist and specialist physicians caring for people living with HIV/AIDS in North Carolina. *Journal of General Internal Medicine, 19*, 16-27.

Goldie, S., Paltiel, D., Weinstein, M., Losina, E., Seage, G., Kimmel, A., Walensky, R., Sax, P., & Freedberg, K. (2003). Projecting the cost-effectiveness of adherence interventions in persons with human immunodeficiency virus infection. *The American Journal of Medicine, 115*, 632-641.

Haubrich, R. H., Little, S. J., Currier, J. S., Forthal, D. N., & Kemper, C. A. (1999). The value of patient-reported adherence to antiretroviral therapy in predicting virologic and immunologic response. *AIDS, 13*, 1099-1107.

Holmberg, S. D. (1996). The estimated prevalence and incidence of HIV in 96 large US metropolitan areas. *American Journal of Public Health, 86*, 642-654.

Holzemer, W. L., Corless, I. B., Nokes, K. M., Turner, J. G., Brown, M. A., Powell-Cope, G. M. et al. (1999). Predictors of self-reported adherence in persons living with HIV disease. *AIDS Patient Care and STDS, 13*, 185-197.

Kalichman, S. C., Ramachandran, B., & Catz, S. (1999). Adherence to Combination Antiretroviral Therapies in HIV Patients of Low Health Literacy. *Journal of General Internal Medicine, 14*, 267-273.

Konkle-Parker, D. J. (2001). A motivational intervention to improve adherence to treatment of chronic disease. *Journal of the American Academy of Nurse Practitioners, 13*, 61-68.

Lucas, G. M., Cheever, L. W., Chaisson, R. E., & Moore, R. D. (2001). Detrimental effects of continued illicit drug use on the treatment of HIV-1 infection. *Journal of Acquired Immune Deficiency Syndromes, 27*, 251-259.

Lyon, M., Trexler, C., Akpan-Townsend, C., Pao, M., Selden, K., Fletcher, J., Addlestone, I., & D'Angelo, L. (2003). A family group therapy approach to increasing adherence to therapy in HIV-infected youths: results of a pilot project. *AIDS Patient Care and STDs, 17*, 299-308.

McPherson-Baker, S., Malow, R., Penedo, F., Jones, D., Schneiderman, N., & Klimas, N. (2000). Enhancing adherence to combination antiretroviral therapy in non-adherent HIV-positive men. *AIDS Care, 12*, 399-404.

Miller, W. R. & Rollnick, S. (2002). *Motivational interviewing, preparing people to change.* (2 ed.) New York: The Guilford Press.

Morgenstern, J., Kahler, C. W., & Epstein, E. (1998). Do treatment process factors mediate the relationship between type A-type B and outcome in 12-Step oriented substance abuse treatment? *Addiction, 93*, 1765-1775.

NYC Department of Health (2003). Quarterly report. *HIV Surveillance and Epidemiology Program, 1(1)*.

Ostrop, N. J., Hallett, K. A., & Gill, M. J. (2000). Long-term patient adherence to antiretroviral therapy. *The Annals of Pharmacotherapy, 34*, 703-709.

Parsons, J. T., Rosof, E., Punzalan, J. C., & DiMaria, L. (2005). Integration of motivational interviewing and cognitive behavioral therapy to improve HIV medication adherence and reduce substance use among HIV-positive men and women: Results of a pilot project. *AIDS Patient Care and STDs, 19*, 31-39.

Patterson, D. L., Swindells, S., Mohr, J., Brester, M., Vergis, E. N., Squire, C. et al. (2000). Adherence to protease inhibitory therapy and outcomes in patients with HIV infection. *Annals of Internal Medicine, 133(1)*, 21-30.

Prochaska, J. O. & DiClemente, C. C. (1992). The transtheoretical approach. In J. C. Norcross & M. R. Goldfried (Eds.), *Handbook of psychotherapy integration* (pp. 300-334). New York: Basic Books.

Rawlings, M. K., Thompson, M. A., Farthing, C. F., Brown, L. S., Racine, J., Scott, R. C., Crawford, K. H., Goodwin, S. D., Tolson, J. M., Williams, V. C., & Schaefer, M. S. (2003). Impact of an educational program on efficacy and adherence with a twice-daily lamivudine/zidovudine/abacavir regimen in underrepresented HIV-infected patients. *Journal of Acquired Immune Deficiency Syndromes, 34(2)*, 174-183.

Reif, S., Smith, S. R., & Golin, C. E. (2003). Medication adherence practices of HIV/AIDS case managers: a statewide survey in North Carolina. *AIDS Patient Care and STDS., 17*, 471-481.

Reynolds, N. R., Testa, M. A., Marc, L. G., Chesney, M. A., Neidig, J. L., Smith, S. R. et al. (2004). Factors influencing medication adherence beliefs and self-efficacy in persons naive to antiretroviral therapy: A multicenter, cross-sectional study. *AIDS and Behavior, 8*, 141-150.

Rigsby, M., Rosen, M., Beauvais, J., Cramer, J., Rainey, P., O'Malley, S., Dieckhause, K., & Rounsaville, B. (2000) Cue-dose training with monetary reinforcement, pilot study of antiretroviral adherence intervention. *Journal of General Internal Medicine, 15*, 841-847.

Roberts, K. & Volberding, P. (1999). Adherence communication: a qualitative analysis of physician-patient dialogue. *AIDS, 13*, 1771-1778.

Safren, S. A., Otto, M. W., Worth, J. L., Salomon, E., Johnson, W., Mayer, K. et al. (2000). Two strategies to increase adherence to HIV antiretroviral medication: Life-steps and medication monitoring. *Behaviour Research and Therapy, 39*, 1151-1162.

Salomon, H., Wainberg, M. A., Brenner, B., Quan, Y., Rouleau, D., Cote, P. et al. (2000). Prevalence of HIV-1 resistant to antiretroviral drugs in 81 individuals newly infected by sexual contact or injecting drug use. *AIDS, 14*, F17-F23.

Samet, J. H., Friedmann, P., & Saitz, R. (2001). Benefits of linking primary medical care and substance abuse services. Patient, Provider, and Societal Perspectives. *Archives of Internal Medicine, 161*, 85-89.

Selwyn, P. A., Budner, N. S., Wasserman, W. C., & Arno, P. S. (1997). Utilization of on-site primary care services by HIV-seropositive and seronegative drug users in a methadone maintenance program. *Public Health Reports, 492*.

Sharpe, T. T., Lee, L. M., Elam-Evans, L. D., & Fleming, P. L. (2004). Crack cocaine use and adherence to antiretroviral treatment among HIV-infected black women. *Journal of Community Health, 29*, 117-127.

Simoni, J., Frick, P., Pantalone, D., & Turner, B. (2003). Antiretroviral adherence interventions: a review of current literature and ongoing studies. *Topics in HIV Medicine, 11*, 185-198.

Sorensen, J. L., Mascovich, A., Wall, T. L., DePhilippis, D., Batki, S. L., & Chesney, M. (1998). Medication adherence strategies for drug abusers with HIV/AIDS. *AIDS Care, 10*, 297-312.

Tucker, J. S., Burnam, M. A., Sherbourne, C. D., & Kung, F. Y. (2003). Substance use and mental health correlates of nonadherence to antiretroviral medications in a sample of patients with human immunodeficiency virus infection. *The American Journal of Medicine, 114*, 573-580.

Tuldra, A., Fumax, C., Ferrer, M., Bayes, R., Arno, A., Balague, M., Bonjoch, A., Jou, A., Negredo, E., Paredes, R., Ruiz, L., Romeu, J., Siera, G., Tural, C., Burger, D., & Clotet, B. (2000). Prospective randomized two-arm controlled study to determine the efficacy of a specific intervention to improve long-term adherence to highly active antiretroviral therapy. *Journal of Acquired Immune Deficiency Syndromes, 25*, 221-228.

Valenti, W. M. (2001). Treatment adherence improves outcomes and manages costs. *AIDS Reader, 11*, 77-80.

Wright, M. T. (2000). The old problem of adherence: research on treatment adherence and its relevance for HIV/AIDS. *AIDS Care, 12*, 703-710.

doi:10.1300/J187v06n01_07

Specialized Adherence Counselors Can Improve Treatment Adherence: Guidelines for Specific Treatment Issues

Teresa L. Scheid, PhD

SUMMARY. Individuals living with HIV disease often have great difficulty adhering to drug treatment regimes. In order to improve treatment adherence clients were referred to a specialized adherence counselor for intensive adherence counseling and education. Instruments were developed which integrated research tools into on-going clinical assessments. The first 30 clients who received adherence counseling were tracked for at least one year in order to assess treatment adherence; 33% were discharged as adherent and 40% exhibited improved adherence; only 10% still had problems with adherence at the 12 month follow-up. This paper describes the role played by specialized adherence counselors and provides a summary of the guidelines that were developed throughout the

Teresa L. Scheid, PhD, is Full Professor in the Department of Sociology, University of North Carolina at Charlotte.

Address correspondence to: Teresa L. Scheid, Department of Sociology, University of North Carolina at Charlotte, 9201 University City Boulevard, Charlotte, NC 28223 (Email: tlscheid@email. uncc.edu).

The author would like to acknowledge the three adherence counselors on this project who worked so hard to help their clients and the useful suggestions for revisions to this paper made by the editors and the reviewers.

Funding for this project was provided by the Regional HIV/AIDS Consortium, Charlotte, NC 28227.

[Haworth co-indexing entry note]: "Specialized Adherence Counselors Can Improve Treatment Adherence: Guidelines for Specific Treatment Issues." Scheid, Teresa L. Co-published simultaneously in *the Journal of HIV/AIDS & Social Services* (The Haworth Press, Inc.) Vol. 6, No. 1/2, 2007, pp. 121-138; and: *HIV Treatment Adherence: Challenges for Social Services* (ed: Lana Sue Ka'opua and Nathan L. Linsk) The Haworth Press, Inc., 2007, pp. 121-138. Single or multiple copies of this article are available for a fee from The Haworth Document Delivery Service [1-800-HAWORTH, 9:00 a.m. - 5:00 p.m. (EST). E-mail address: docdelivery@haworthpress.com].

121

course of this project. Strategies are offered for helping with diverse adherence problems describing how "to do" adherence counseling directed towards clinicians working on the front line to improve adherence.

doi:10.1300/J187v06n01_08 *[Article copies available for a fee from The Haworth Document Delivery Service: 1-800-HAWORTH. E-mail address: <docdelivery@ haworthpress.com> Website: <http://www.HaworthPress.com> © 2007 by The Haworth Press, Inc. All rights reserved.]*

KEYWORDS. Adherence, adherence counselors, clinician role, HIV/ AIDS

INTRODUCTION

Human Immunodeficiency Virus (HIV) is a highly infectious disease that is transmitted mainly through unprotected sex, intravenous drug use, or passed from mother to fetus. HIV is a virus that breaks down a person's immune system, or CD-4 cells, which is the system that fights diseases (Department of Health and Human Services [DHHS], 2003). The amount of HIV virus in the body is assessed by examining the viral load in the blood (DHHS). Antiretroviral drugs reduce the viral load both by attacking the virus and inhibiting the virus from reproducing, allowing people with HIV disease to live longer and healthier lives. Antiretroviral drugs, when successful, reduce the viral load in the blood and increase the CD-4 counts. However, in order to be effective these drugs must be taken properly. Antiretroviral drugs have complicated dosing regimes; they must be taken at certain times, with or without food, and have many side effects. To reduce the viral load, treatment guidelines specify that antiretroviral drugs must be taken correctly at least 95% of the time (DHHS). The costs of non-adherence are serious; the virus can mutate and become drug resistant. This is especially likely with the combinations of non-nucleoside reverse transcriptase inhibitors (NNRTIs or non-nukes) and Protease Inhibitors. Drug resistant strains of HIV place the individual at an increased risk of death and also pose a larger public health threat (DHHS). As Demmer (2003) notes, regular assessment of treatment adherence is critical and health care providers need to be involved in the development and evaluation of interventions designed to improve adherence.

This paper describes a unique program, which utilized specialized adherence counselors to assist clients with adherence problems. The author served as the evaluator for the project and tracked clients referred to the program during the first year for at least one year; adherence improved for 73% of the clients who received counseling. At the completion of the evaluation of the project the author, in consultation with the adherence counselors, developed a treatment adherence manual that is user-friendly and synthesizes what is known about treatment adherence with the experiences of the adherence counselors, giving concrete, practical suggestions for improving adherence in their clients. During the past year we have revised the manual several times and used it in adherence workshops for HIV case managers and to train newly hired adherence counselors. After briefly describing our study and its main findings, I present a summary of the materials in the treatment manual in the hopes that the guidelines we have developed will be of use to others seeking to assist clients with treatment adherence. This paper is motivated by the fact that the adherence counselors could find very little guidance in the literature on how "to do" adherence counseling, and it is directed towards clinicians working on the front line to address various types of adherence problems their clients face.

BACKGROUND AND SIGNIFICANCE

There is a tremendous amount of literature reviewing factors associated with patient adherence to antiretroviral medications (for example, Catz, Kelly, Bogard, Benotsch, & McAuliffe, 2000; Cook et al., 2002; Fogarty et al., 2002; Powell-Cope, White, Henkelman, Turner, & Haley, 2003; Safren et al., 2001; Schilder et al., 2001; Tucker, Burnam, Sherbourne, Jung, & Gilford, 2003; Wainberg & Cournos, 2000). Later in this paper I will provide a brief summary of the major factors associated with adherence and non-adherence. This review focuses on literature which addresses how provider based interventions can improve adherence.

The clinicians hired as adherence counselors for this project searched for specific guidance on how to perform their roles, and we found very little literature on how providers can effectively improve adherence. Brook et al. (2001) report that continuing support from specific health care workers encouraged adherence. Safren et al. (2001) found that motivational interviewing and a problem solving session led to improved adherence for persons with adherence problems. Kalichman et al. (2001) also found that motivational interviewing significantly reduced the number of doses missed. Wainberg and Cournos (2000) report on the effectiveness of mental health counseling. Controlled studies of counseling and education by nurses (Pradier et al., 2002) and pharmacists (Haddad et al., 2002) have found these health care providers to be effective in promoting adherence.

Adherence is also associated with good relationships with physicians (Roberts, 2000), although Golin, Smith, and Reif (2004) found that physicians need more training and time to provide adherence counseling to their patients. Likewise, pharmacists often do not have enough time to provide adherence counseling (Smith, Golin, & Reif, 2004). Reif, Smith and Golin (2003) found that the majority of HIV case managers surveyed in North Carolina did feel adherence counseling was part of their role, although a third did not feel they had adequate training to provide such counseling. Given the dearth of available treatment staff to monitor patient adherence, Broadhead et al. (2002) developed a peer-driven intervention to provide alternative forms of social support for active drug users with HIV infection. Molassiotis, Lopex-Has, Chung, and Lam (2003) report on the success of a three-month patient education model with individualized weekly counseling and follow-up telephone calls. They recommend that clients be supported with individualized management programs, which was the purpose of the adherence counseling model utilized in this study.

DESCRIPTION OF THE STUDY

The local Regional HIV/AIDS Consortium serves a 13 county region in North Carolina and secured funding to hire three adherence counselors; two counselors were nurses and one was a social worker; two were white women and one was a Black male. One adherence counselor, the social worker, did only adherence counseling while the other two worked part-time as adherence counselors. Several months were spent learning the newest information about HIV medications and adherence. Over the course of the first year, adherence counselors and the evaluator continued to meet monthly to develop strategies for improving adherence. In an effort to evaluate the effectiveness of specialized adherence counseling, instruments were developed that integrated research tools into on-going clinical assessments.

First, an adherence referral form for use by doctors, nurses, or case managers was developed. Once referred, adherence counselors completed an intake interview that assessed the client's living situation, treatment history, sources of social support, co-occurring health problems, substance use, mental illness, and medical history. If the client had been taking antiretroviral drugs, a five-day medication recall history was completed. Adherence counselors also completed a 56-item treatment barriers checklist (Catz et al. 2000) to help them determine existing or potential sources of non-adherence. Adherence counselors noted that clients' reasons for non-adherence were often not those commonly assessed by shorter scales; they also found that completion of the treatment barriers checklist helped them to know their clients better. Sample items included:

- Treatment interferes with time I spend with family and friends.
- I have too many other things to do.
- I don't want to change what I do every day.
- I don't feel comfortable talking to doctors.
- It is hard to plan meals around taking medicine.
- I don't have a good way to keep track of time.

Three-month progress notes were completed to assess adherence, to note any existing problems or concerns, and to describe any changes in the client's living situation. Adherence counselors also noted specific barriers to adherence, as well as clients' strengths relative to adherence.

During the first year of the program, 53 clients were referred for adherence counseling. Of these, 11 were not seen after the initial intake and could not be contacted despite repeated efforts by adherence counselors. Of the 42 seen for continued adherence counseling, five were never placed on HAART and another five died while two moved out of the service area. Thirty clients were on antiretroviral drugs and received adherence counseling for at least one year in order to address problems with adherence. The majority of these clients were male (70%, n = 21) and African American (83.3%, n = 25). They were equally from urban, suburban, and rural areas (two adherence counselors served rural and suburban areas while the third served a larger metropolitan area). All clients were poor and receiving Ryan White funding for services. The majority lacked stable social support systems, though they all had case-managers who helped them meet their multiple needs.

Adherence was assessed by three measures: client self report, clinician assessment and lab work. All three measures of adherence had to concur in adherence for improvement to be noted. That is, if laboratory work, self report, and clinician appraisal all indicated improvement in adherence at the three-month progress report, adherence was assessed as improved. Important to clinician assessment of adherence was refill history as assessed by either direct observation factors such as client brings medications to the clinic, clinician fills prescriptions, or fills pill boxes for the client, or verification by the pharmacist that prescriptions had been refilled when feasible. Non-adherence was indicated if client self reported missing doses, or if clinician had any reason to believe client was not fully adherent by either objective evidence such as doses not taken, or subjective feeling that client was not being honest about adherence, or if lab work showed regression. Clients were discharged from the program when they had been assessed as fully adherent with no missed doses for six months verified through at least two three month progress reports. In addition, clinicians also checked with their clients six months after discharge to determine if they were still adherent.

RESULTS

Table 1 compares the six- and 12-month adherence outcomes for these 30 clients. As can be seen, adherence steadily improved for clients with 57% (17) showing improved adherence at the six-month follow-up, and 33% (10) discharged adherent at the 12-month follow-up. Seventeen percent (5) were non-adherent at the six-month follow-up and ten percent (3) were still non-adherent at the 12-month follow-up. Four clients had been taken off antiretroviral drugs between the six and 12-month follow-up as their lab work indicated some problems or because of co-occurring health problems. We found that there is a need for ongoing and long-term follow-up in order to improve adherence, and some clients who were still not adherent at the 12-month follow-up did eventually show signs of improvement.

TABLE 1. Six- and 12-Month Outcomes for Recipients of Adherence Counseling (n = 30)

Client Adherence	6 Month		12 Month	
	n	%	N	%
Working to Improve Adherence	7	23	1	3
Improved Adherence	17	57	12	40
Discharged Adherent	1	3	10	33
Not Adherent	5	17	3	10
Taken off HAART	0	–	4	13
Totals	30	100	30	99

LESSONS LEARNED

The strategies and frameworks that we found to be most helpful in helping clients improve their adherence were utilized to create adherence guidelines, which we have used in training workshops for HIV case managers and newly hired specialized adherence counselors. While the November 2003 DHHS, "Guidelines for the Use of Antiretroviral Agents" is very thorough, the adherence counselors wanted a more concise "how to" manual to help them quickly identify adherence problems and which specified what types of actions on their part would be most effective in addressing that client's non-adherence. Drawing upon some of the practice oriented research literature on adherence, and the experiences of counselors in this project, in the following sections I very briefly identify those factors the adherence counselors found to be most salient in understanding adherence and non-adherence.

Understanding Non-Adherence

The DHHS "Guidelines for use of Antiretroviral Agents" (November 2003: 10) provides a thorough summary of the scholarly literature and identifies the following factors as major sources of non-adherence:

1. Lack of trust between clinician and client
2. Active drug and alcohol use
3. Active mental illness or depression
4. Lack of patient education and inability of clients to identify medication
5. Lack of reliable access to primary medical care or medications
6. Side effects.

In relation to these guidelines we found that adherence counselors are successful to the degree that they develop a good relationship with their clients, especially when the former provide ongoing positive reinforcement and social support. Specifically adherence counselors:

- Work to increase client's understanding of their illness and the need to take medications as prescribed.
- Help clients to find techniques to cope with the side effects, and monitor the degree to which side effects result in non-adherence.
- Assist clients in gaining access to medication through drug assistance programs or other sources, including patient assistance through drug companies.

- Assess problems with substance use, and discuss with physicians whether medications should be withheld until the client has committed to substance abuse treatment.
- Attend to client's mental condition. Many individuals with HIV disease experience depression and stress, and these are major factors to consider in beginning a treatment regime or enhancing adherence.

In addition to the factors identified by the DHHS (2003), a major barrier to adherence is client denial of the illness (Whetten-Goldstein & Nguyen, 2002). Medication adherence is a daily reminder of the illness, and a common response to any chronic illness is denial. HIV disease is also highly stigmatizing, and clients are reluctant to disclose their status for fear of discrimination and negative evaluations from family and friends. Consequently, the degree to which a client has accepted their HIV status, and has the support of family and/or friends are critical factors in adherence. Clients are also less likely to take their medications when they are feeling well and therefore, feel as though they do not need medication, and the same occurs if they feel sick and the medications make them feel sicker. Adherence counselors must monitor adherence over a long period of time to help clients through these various stages in learning to live with HIV disease and a potentially difficult medication regimen.

Another source of non-adherence is that the patient simply forgets, or has trouble fitting the medication into their daily routine. This may be due to work, travel, sleep and eating patterns, being too busy, or other factors relevant to the client's lifestyle. Adherence counselors help clients find ways to fit medications into their daily routine, and introduce clients to the use of pill boxes, alarms, or various reminder systems to help them remember to take their medications. Eliciting support from family or friends, or other social supports can help improve adherence in these cases.

Sources of Adherence

The DHHS Guidelines (2003: 10) identify the major predictors of optimal adherence as:

1. Emotional and practical life supports
2. Ability to fit medications in daily routine
3. Understanding that non-adherence leads to treatment resistance

4. Recognition that taking all medication doses as prescribed is critical
5. Feeling comfortable taking medication in front of people. This indicates acceptance of the illness.
6. Keeping clinical appointments.

We have found that adherence is enhanced when clients express a "will to live" and are ready to work to live with the disease. Often spiritual beliefs are critical to developing a will to live. Once the client is committed to treatment, the adherence counselor can help educate the client and teach them the importance of taking medications as prescribed and to understand how the medications work.

Assessment of client adherence is an important issue for the clinician. We have found that using a short-term assessment of medication taken in the recent past (3 to 5 days) and identification of common treatment barriers are helpful in assessing treatment adherence. Having clients bring their medications or medication diaries to clinic visits can be helpful, as can checking with the pharmacist to see if prescriptions have been refilled on schedule. We have found that home visits are essential, because the clinician can see where medications are kept and assess those factors, which prevent optimal adherence. Many clients need to have an adherence counselor fill their pillboxes on a weekly or bi-weekly basis. Other clients needed to have the adherence counselor actually fill the prescription for them.

While the DHHS Guidelines (2003) have been useful in beginning to think about adherence, we found that the adherence counselors wanted more specific guidance on differential adherence strategies for use with diverse adherence problems. The following guidelines are based upon the adherence counselor's experiences with a number of different clients and adherence problems.

CLIENT SPECIFIC ADHERENCE STRATEGIES

After two years of working with clients with adherence problems and ongoing literature review, we decided to codify the practices that seemed to work and to develop guidelines which would help other providers (i.e., case managers, nurses, and social workers) improve treatment adherence. We have found that different strategies work with clients at different stages of treatment readiness and the following guidelines identify critical components of the provider role for clients at each stage. Table 2 provides a summary of these guidelines.

TABLE 2. Summary of Client Specific Adherence Strategies

Client Stage	Source of Non-Adherence	Counselor's Role	Strategy
Newly Diagnosed	Denial of Illness and Stigma	Be a Friend Establish trust	Demonstrate positive regard and acceptance of client
Starting HAART	Lack of Patient Education and Knowledge	Teach Client, Advocate	Education Regular Planned Contact
On HAART	Perceptions and Beliefs	Partner	Continued Contact
On HAART, Not Adherent	Problems with Life Depression, Anxiety, Substance Abuse	Empower Client	1. Address specific client barriers to adherence. 2. Refer to multi-disciplinary team for discussion.

Recently Diagnosed Clients

When clients have recently been diagnosed, there will in all likelihood be a period of denial, followed by anger, depression and guilt. Most clients at this stage either do not accept their illnesses, or do not want to take medication that reminds them of their illness. Since they have not yet accepted the reality of their illness, they will not actively seek out support or treatment, and the stigmatizing effects of HIV/AIDS are most powerful at this time. One of the most damaging consequences of stigma is that individuals internalize the stigmatizing labels, and suffer lower self-esteem and demoralization. Due to these identified emotional states, factors our counselors found critical to adherence are:

• A good relationship with a healthcare provider/case manager–the client must know you care
• Self-esteem and acceptance of the illness label
• Good social support

The provider's role is to establish trust. The provider is available to listen to concerns empathically and may call regularly and spend time with them like a friend, as well as help problem solve to maintain good adherence. They may not have anyone else to talk to about their HIV status. Home visits, lunch, coffee, frequent telephone contact are all important strategies to build trust.

Client Indicates Readiness to Initiate HAART

At this point, the client has accepted their illness, and feels ready to begin treatment. This is the time for intensive education, in the form of handouts or videos. If the client has limited reading skills (and most high school graduates read at the 8th grade level), use videos. Look for handouts that are user friendly, with pictures and large captions. Education should take place in stages, with small amounts of information given at each session. Education should continue for a number of weeks, each time asking the client to tell you what they "know" (a refresher from the last education session), and what questions they have about the material covered; then you can proceed with new information. The basic components of HIV Patient Education include the following as identified in the DHHS Guidelines (2003):

- Basic pathophysiology of HIV infection
- Purpose and goals of antiretrovirals
- Duration of therapy and administration schedule
- Potential side effects and suggested responses to deal with the side effects
- Concept of resistance and importance of adherence to medication regime
- Potential for drug-drug interactions and important food-drug interactions

Arrange to visit a physician and a pharmacist with the client, and discuss the client's overall health needs, other medications, history of compliance or non-compliance with other medications, best time to take medications, number of pills that can be handled at one time. With both the physician and the patient, discuss the best antiretroviral regime (and so far there is not scientific evidence that points to optimal regimes) for that client. One size does not fit all, and you will have to play the role of advocate for the client in his/her conversations with the doctor or pharmacist. Clients are often disenfranchised and are not likely to voice their concerns or to ask questions.

The provider role is that of teacher and to some degree, advocate. Weekly sessions on HIV 101 should be conducted until the client has a good understanding of the illness and of the needs for medications and the importance of taking 95% of their doses (for a once-a-day regime this is taking 29 out of 30 days, rather than a missed morning or two evenings with a twice-a-day regime).

Helping Clients Already on HAART

The following factors have been identified as critical to patient's decisions to maintain their medications and continue adhering to treatment (Whetten-Goldstein & Nguyen, 2002). Be sure to address the client's perceptions and beliefs.

- Trust in the healthcare system: good experiences with doctors and other providers, feeling that confidentiality is protected, and does not believe in conspiracy theory.
- Perceived seriousness of the disease
- Perceived susceptibility to future health declines (i.e., it will get better, or worse).
- Perceived benefits of services and treatment
- Perceived value client's support system places on services and treatment
- Perceived ability to use services, to adhere to treatment.

Work with the client to alter perceptions if necessary. Adherence is increased with higher levels of self-esteem, self-efficacy, and when the client feels they have some control. Most individuals are initially compliant with HAART (for three months) and then adherence drops, which is referred to as pill fatigue in the DHHS Guidelines (2003). Even when clients have demonstrated adherence, be sure and monitor the impact of new diagnoses or co-morbidities such as depression, liver disease, other health problems, continued or recurring substance abuse on adherence and assess every 6 months for fully adherent clients. Contact should be made every 3 months or more frequently for those with continuing adherence problems. Intensify management efforts during periods of low adherence with increased visits, use of other team members, and referrals to mental health or substance abuse services.

The provider's role is one of partner. Once the client has begun HAART, call a number of times the first week, then call weekly to check on problems or questions for one month, and then check with the client at least once a month for 6 months to be sure they remain compliant and do not experience complications or drug interactions. We have found home visits to be particular useful. Lab work results should be shared with the client so they can then see the gains that are made. Alternatively, if gains are not evident, changes in the medication may be necessary. Do not assume non-adherence; if you have established a good relationship with the client, they will most likely be truthful about their adherence.

Client Has Difficulty with HAART

Based upon our experience, providers first need to discover the source of the non-adherence; then a response can be formulated. The major sources of client non-adherence followed by effective provider response are:

1. Client feels medications remind them of their illness, or they must hide evidence of medications from family/friends/co-workers.
    Provider must work on acceptance of the illness with this client and help the client in facing the reality of stigma.
2. Client has experienced side effects and/or has other medications, which may have interacted with HAART medications. Often the client feels sicker on medications. Almost everyone experiences side effects, and the distress they cause should not be minimized. Some side effects may be life-threatening.
    Provider must be familiar with the typical as well as the atypical side effects of the medications their client is taking, and be pre-pared to consult with the doctor or pharmacist if side effects are serious or are interfering with adherence. The provider must be understanding and work with the client to reduce common side ef-fects, as well as the discomfort from symptoms such as diarrhea. Letting clients know side effects will subside, and providing client with specific knowledge and resources to deal with side ef-fects/symptoms both provides comfort to the client and empower-ment that they have learned strategies to make themselves feel better. There are a number of client education sheets and booklets the adherence counselors utilized, which provided detailed and thorough suggestions for dealing with various side effects of med-ication and consequences of the illness. Many of these handouts are available through pharmaceutical companies or via the web. It is important that the adherence counselor deal with each client as an individual and seek individual solutions to common problems (for example, avoiding some foods when experiencing diarrhea or eating more of those foods which help prevent diarrhea).
3. Client forgets to take medications. Most people are not adherent to their medications; we all self medicate in that we take what we feel we need, when we feel we need it.

Provider: Patient education is critical for these clients, and must be ongoing. Client's perceptions may need to change, so that s/he understands the medications have value. Clients should be empowered, by for example teaching them how to keep track of their lab results, so they can see the positive gains associated with their medications. Furthermore, clients need to be reminded that everyone will occasionally forget to take their medications. Pill fatigue is a common experience in HIV care, where adherence decreases for even the most adherent clients. Providers must work with the client and determine which mechanisms will help them remember to take their medications. Adherence counselors utilized all of the following mechanisms and strategies with clients: pill boxes, alarms, refilling prescriptions for the client, filling pill boxes weekly, home visits, creation of social support such as a friend or family member calls the client, and linking e client to support groups. If necessary, providers can create such support groups as they did in this project. Support groups are among the most powerful tool for changing behavior and enforcing compliance (Broadhead et al., 2002). Peer support is especially valuable, as is having a consumer advocate.

4. Client may have problems in their life such as depression, instability in income, housing, work, and lack of supports. Both stress and depression interfere with adherence, and also weaken the immune system.

   Providers should not encourage clients to begin antiretroviral treatment until the client has a stable way to pay for the medications, which does not interfere with their need to buy food or pay for housing. Clients should be linked to a case manager and to other needed social supports and resources. Linkages to mental health counseling, and other social supports, unfortunately may take time, but can be instrumental in promoting adherence.

5. Client has substance abuse problems. This is probably the most difficult situation to deal with. Many physicians do not feel a client should take antiretroviral medication if they are abusing substances; however, substance use is often a way of dealing with the depression associated with a HIV diagnosis, or may be part of the client's environment and perhaps injection was the cause for HIV transmission.

   Providers should support their client's efforts to engage in less risky behavior. The DHHS (2003) adherence treatment guidelines support harm reduction, which moves the client towards abstinence by allowing for occasional relapses. Clients needing additional support to address their substance use problems should be referred to a substance abuse professional, treatment program and/or support groups such as Alcoholics Annonymous, Cocaine Annonymous, or Narcotics Annonymous.

The provider role is to empower clients, and become familiar with the client's case history, and circumstances in their life, which will work for, or against adherence. Clinicians must learn to recognize that each client is unique, and faces a number of problems in their day-to-day life. Home visits were critical components to the adherence counseling provided in this project. Home visits helped the counselor to understand the client and their life situation, and also told the client that the counselor really cared about them. Through such personal contact counselors avoided being perceived by clients as the "medication police." Many clients simply needed someone to stop by on a regular basis and care about their well-being and/or help them to fill their prescriptions and pill boxes.

IMPLICATIONS FOR SOCIAL SERVICES

This paper describes a program of specialized adherence counseling and follow-up. We found that adherence counseling was successful in that over 70% (21) of the clients who received such counseling demonstrated improved adherence. In this study eleven of the 53-referred clients with adherence problems were unwilling/unable to meet with an adherence counselor and these clients are also probably more likely not to be receiving continuing preventative health care for their HIV. None of these clients were receiving services at the 12-month follow up. Devising an improved intervention that would retain this most difficult client population would require further study to examine the nature of this population, and follow-up to determine their reasons for not returning. In the meantime it means that provider must work hard to make meaningful contact with clients at the very first visit, stressing that HIV medication and treatment adherence are both long-term projects.

Because so many clients fail to follow through with medical appointments as well as medication, the most important factor in the success of our adherence program was that counselors went to client's homes rather than relying upon office-based visits. Clinic appointments can place the provider in a more powerful position relative to the client and may mitigate the feeling of trust that is critical to adherence. Home visits also allow the adherence counselor to see where medications are kept and to assess factors which contribute to non-adherence.

Adherence counseling, as found in our study, is effective and does lead to improved adherence. Consequently, adherence counseling should be considered as a critical component to HIV disease management, but we found there is a need for long term follow-up and continued patient education in order to fully address non-adherence. Because of the need for continued support, adherence counseling should be considered an essential component of the HIV case manager role, many of whom are social workers. We found that the ultimate key to the success of our program was developing an open, trusting relationship with clients and providing positive, not negative reinforcement.

Crucial to adherence is acceptance of the illness, understanding of the role of medications, and a positive sense that taking medication will help. Adherence counselors helped clients gain that sense of mastery and also helped them cope with the stigma of HIV disease. Adherence counselors were also an important source of social support for clients who had very few other resources. Obviously adherence counseling is not a quick fix; but we found adherence is not simply a medical issue. Instead, adherence involves the full spectrum of an individual's life and belief system and changing these to improve adherence will take follow-up, not just a one patient education session. We hope that the strategies and guidelines outlined in this paper have provided useful ideas to help our colleagues working to improve the health of their clients through treatment and medication adherence.

REFERENCES

Broadhead, R. S., Heckathorn, D. D. Altice, F. L., Hulst, Y., Carbone, M., Friedland, G. H. et al. (2002). Increasing drug users' adherence to HIV treatment: Results of a peer-driven intervention feasibility study. *Social Science & Medicine, 55*, 235-46.

Brook, M. G., Dale, A., Tomlinson, D., Waterworth, C., Daniels, D., & Forster, G. (2001). Adherence to highly active antiretroviral therapy in the real world: Experience of twelve English HIV units. *AIDS Patient Care and STDs, 15*(9), 491-4.

Catz, S. L., Kelly, J. A., Bogard, L. M., Benotsch, E. G., & McAuliffe, T. L. (2000). Patterns, correlates, and barriers to medication adherence among persons prescribed new treatments for HIV disease. *Health Psychology, 19*(2), 124-33.

Cook, J. A., Cohen, M. H., Burke, J., Grey, D., Anastos, K., Kirstein, L. et al. (2002). Effects of depressive symptoms and mental health quality of life on use of highly active antiretroviral therapy among HIV-seropositive women. *Journal of Acquired Immune Deficiency 30*(4), 401-9.

Demmer, C. (2003). Treatment adherence among clients in AIDS service organizations. *Journal of HIV/AIDS & Social Services, 2*(3), 33-47.

Department of Health and Human Services. (2003). Guidelines for the use of antiretroviral agents in HIV-1-infected adults and adolescents. Retrieved on November 10, 2003 at http://AIDSinfo.nih.gov A more recent (2005) version is available.

Fogarty, L., Roter, D., Larson, S., Burke, J., Gillespie, J., & Levy, R. (2002). Patient adherence to HIV medication regimes: A review of published and abstract reports. *Patient Education Counseling, 46*(2) 93-108.

Golin, C. E., Smith, S., & Reif, S. (2004). Practices of generalist and specialist physicians caring for people living with HIV/AIDS in North Carolina. *Journal of General Internal Medicine, 19*(1), 16-27.

Haddad, M., Inch, C., Glazier, R. H., Wilkins, A. L., Urbshott, G. B., Bayoumi, A. et al. (2002). Patient support and education for promoting adherence to highly active antiretroviral therapy for HIV/AIDS. Cochrane Review, *The Cochrane Library, 1*, 2002. Retrieved from Medscape, 3/19/2002.

Kalichman, S. C., Rompa, D., DiFonzo, K., Simpson, D. I., Austin, J., Luke, W. et al. (2001). HIV treatment adherence in women living with HIV/AIDS: Research based on the Information-Motivation-Behavioral Skills model of health behavior. *Journal of the Association of Nurses in AIDS Care, 12*(4), 58-67.

Molossiotis, A., Lopex-Hahas, V., Chung, W. Y., & Lam, S. W. (2003). A pilot study of the effects of a behavioral intervention on treatment adherence in HIV-infected patients. *AIDS Care, 15*(1), 125-35.

Powell-Cope, G. M., White, J., Henkelman, E. J., Turner, B. J., & Haley, J. A. (2003). Qualitative and quantitative assessments of HAART adherence of substance-abusing women. *AIDS Care, 15*(2), 239-49.

Pradier, C., Bentz, L., Spire, B., Tourette-Turgis, C., Morin, M., Fuzibet, J. et al. (2002). Adherence to therapy, 9th conference on retroviruses and opportunistic infection, Session 73. February 24-28, Seattle, Washington.

Reif, S., Smith, S., & Golin, C. E. (2003), Medication adherence practices of HIV/AIDS case managers: A statewide survey in North Carolina. *AIDS Patient Care and STDs, 17*(9), 471-81.

Roberts, K.J. (2000). Physician beliefs about antiretroviral adherence communication. *AIDS Patient Care & STDs, 14*(9), 477-84.

Safren, S. A., Otto, M. W., Worth, J. L., Salomon, E., Johnson, E., Mayer, K. et al. (2001). Two strategies to increase adherence to HIV antiretroviral medication: Lifesteps and medication monitoring. *Behavior Research and Therapy, 39*(10), 1151-62.

Schilder, A. J., Kennedy, C., Goldstone, I. L., Ogden, R. D., Hogg, R. S., & O'Shaughnessy, M.V. (2001). "Being dealt with as a whole person": Care seeking and adherence: The benefits of culturally competent care. *Social Science & Medicine 52*(11), 1643-59.

Smith, S. R., Golin, C. E., & Reif, S. (2004). Influence of time stress and other variables on counseling by pharmacists about antiretroviral medications. *American Journal of Health-System Pharmacy, 61*(1), 1120-1129.

Tucker, J. S., Burnam, M. A., Sherbourne, C. D., Jung, F. Y., & Gifford, A. L. (2003). Substance use and mental health correlates of non-adherence to antiretroviral medications in a sample of patients with HIV infection. *American Journal of Medicine, 114*(7), 573-80.

Wainberg, M. L. & Cournos, F. (2000). Adherence to treatment. *New Directions in Mental Health Services, 87*, 85-93.

Whetten-Goldstein, K., & Nguyen, T. Q. (2002). *You're the first one I've told: New faces of HIV in the South.* New Brunswick, New Jersey: Rutgers University Press.

doi:10.1300/J187v06n01_08

Training Substance Abuse Counselors About HIV Medication Adherence

Michael Bass, MA, ACSW, CRADC
Nathan L. Linsk, PhD, ACSW
Christopher Mitchell, PhD

SUMMARY. High levels of medication adherence are crucial to the success of HIV treatment. Consequently, substance abuse counselors (SACs), social service and other care providers can best support their HIV positive clients when they understand adherence and related interventions. This paper describes a training program that was designed to increase counselor knowledge of HIV medications, adherence strategies and enhance counseling skills specific to HIV adherence. For substance abuse counselors the training needs included: better understanding of

Michael Bass, MA, ACSW, CRADC, is a doctoral student at the Jane Addams College of Social Work, and Technology Transfer Specialist with the Great Lake Addiction Technology Transfer Center, both at the University of Illinois at Chicago.

Nathan L. Linsk, PhD, ACSW, is Professor at the Jane Addams College of Social Work at the University of Illinois at Chicago. He is Principal Investigator of the Midwest AIDS Training and Education Center and Co-Principal Investigator of the Great Lakes Addiction Technology Transfer Center.

Christopher Mitchell, PhD, is Associate Professor at the Jane Addams College of Social Work where he is Director of the Doctoral Program.

Address correspondence to: Michael Bass, Jane Addams College of Social Work at the University of Illinois at Chicago, 1040 West Harrison, Room 4256 (M/C 309), Chicago, IL 60607 (E-Mail: mikebass@uic.edu).

[Haworth co-indexing entry note]: "Training Substance Abuse Counselors About HIV Medication Adherence." Bass, Michael, Nathan L. Linsk, and Christopher Mitchell. Co-published simultaneously in *the Journal of HIV/AIDS & Social Services* (The Haworth Press, Inc.) Vol. 6, No. 1/2, 2007, pp. 139-159; and: *HIV Treatment Adherence: Challenges for Social Services* (ed: Lana Sue Ka'opua and Nathan L. Linsk) The Haworth Press, Inc., 2007, pp. 139-159. Single or multiple copies of this article are available for a fee from The Haworth Document Delivery Service [1-800-HAWORTH, 9:00 a.m. - 5:00 p.m. (EST). E-mail address: docdelivery@haworthpress.com].

medication interactions, relapse, recovery, and interdisciplinary communication. Thirty-six SACs from three agencies completed the 1 1/2-day
training, which included lecture discussions, case discussion and interac-
tive client case simulations. Success in accomplishing training objectives
was evaluated at three points: pre-intervention training, post-intervention,
and six month follow-up to determine changes in participants' knowledge, attitudes and behaviors related to adherence counseling. Three case
scenarios measuring counselor comfort levels indicated SACs felt significantly more comfortable discussing relapse and medication issues
with their HIV affected clients than they would in discussing medication
issues with the client's physician. However, they felt slightly more
comfortable about physician discussions after training. Open-ended
comments by SACs at six-month follow-up provided insights into recovery issues their clients faced. The findings suggest ways medication
adherence could fit the reality of serving clients with co-occurring
HIV and substance use to better meet their health and support needs.

doi:10.1300/J187v06n01_09 *[Article copies available for a fee from The
Haworth Document Delivery Service: 1-800-HAWORTH. E-mail address:
<docdelivery@haworthpress.com> Website: <http://www.HaworthPress.com>
© 2007 by The Haworth Press, Inc. All rights reserved.]*

KEYWORDS. HIV/AIDS, medication adherence, stages of change,
substance abuse, substance abuse treatment, provider education, training,
client simulation

INTRODUCTION

Challenges for HIV affected clients and providers in successfully
using highly active antiretroviral therapy (HAART) include access to
medication and care, treatment and social support to achieve adherence
necessary for positive outcomes. Specific training models to prepare
providers to help their clients address these challenges, however, are
seldom evaluated. To enhance HIV medication adherence, health and
social service providers require training about HIV medications, effective counseling and other social and educational interventions to ensure
their clients are well informed before taking these medications and that
those taking them will do so on time and without fail. Although required
adherence levels may vary across regimens, the criteria for successful
adherence has been established at 95% of doses to ensure treatment

effectiveness, avoid resistance to the drugs and/or limiting future treatment options, and to avoid transmission of resistant virus to others (Carpenter et al., 2000; Paterson et al., 1999).

Studies have shown that HIV seropositive clients have difficulty changing their behavior to become adherent to medication (Bangsberg, Hecht et al., 2000). In this study we address concerns co-occurring HIV and substance use, which may add a barrier to decision-making about starting these powerful medications, and remaining adherent once HAART has began. Few supports are available for this hard to reach population (Cunningham & Selwyn, 2005; Frank & Miramontes, 1999; Johnson et al., 2003; Lucas, Gebo, Chaisson, & Moore, 2002; Sherer, 1998).

This study was designed to evaluate the impacts of an HIV medication adherence educational program delivered to substance abuse counselors. The evaluation goal was to determine whether there would be attitude and practice changes associated with the training. The following aims were addressed in this project: (1) Extend adherence education to the social service community by educating substance abuse counselors about HIV and HIV medication; (2) Encourage counselors to discuss medication adherence with their clients; and (3) Encourage counselors to discuss medication adherence with their clients' physicians. Evaluation questions included:

1. What was viewed as most useful in the training to address needs of the substance abuse counselors?
2. How comfortable were the participants in addressing medication adherence issues with their HIV positive clients and their health providers?
3. Were there changes in practice patterns associated with this training?

LITERATURE REVIEW

Substance Abuse Co-Occurring with HIV and HAART

Substance use is often viewed as a co-occurring condition with HIV, because of the risk for transmission through injection drug use. Even with the advent of HAART medications, persons affected with HIV who used substances often did not have access to the medication and were often not thought to be a good risk to take these medications regularly (Cunningham & Selwyn, 2005; Sollitto, Mehlman, Youngner, &

Lederman, 2001). However, with the greater availability of medications and the evident health benefits, substance use and HIV are now viewed as conditions that can be treated concurrently (Batki & Selwyn, 2002; Centers for Disease Control and Prevention [CDC], 1998; Paterson et al., 1999; Stein et al., 2000; Ware, Wyatt, & Tugenberg, 2005). It has been noted that medical practitioners, drug companies, AIDS advocates and drug treatment workers have all questioned the suitability of HIV treatment for clients who are "deemed less likely to adhere, [however this is] a dangerous process that can lead to discrimination" (Barthwell, 1997, p. 2, see also Ware et al., 2005).

Earlier studies pointed out an association between availability and use of HIV treatment by race, gender and injection drug use status. Chaisson, Keruly, and Moore (1995) measured disease progression and survival in 1372 HIV positive patients. They found no relation between disease progression and sex, race, injection drug use, income, level of education or insurance status. However, since "57% of all AIDS cases among women have been attributed to injection drug use or sex partners who inject drugs, compared with 31% of cases among men," and mother to infant transmission contribute to 1% of all intravenous drug use (IDU) related transmissions (CDC, 2002, p. 3), the challenge of determining effective outcomes of HAART adherence interventions for those with co-occurring substance-use continues to be compelling. A more recent report by Health Resources and Human Services Administration (HRSA) in 2005 indicates that the number of cases of persons living with AIDS contracted through IDU are 22% for men and 35% for women and that this is a proportion that has continued to decline over the past decade. IDU's have experienced a lower rate (7%) of mortality reduction, than men who have sex with men (15.5%). Of concern is that women whose transmission was via IDU experienced an increase in mortality of 4.4% (HRSA).

Ware et al. (2005) studied adherence patterns of 52 active drug users and found that though many led "chaotic lives," this did not always affect their adherence to HIV medication. They found that many barriers to adherence these individuals faced were similar to ones that non-drug users face. Based on the extant literature on adherence, HIV medication is not precluded from being considered for persons with substance abuse, homelessness and/or psychiatric illness even though it is recognized that it may present some barriers (Bamberger et al., 2000; Bangsberg et al., 2000; Bangsberg, Tulsky, Hecht, & Moss, 1997; Chesney, 2000).

Ancillary Provider Involvement

Despite the co-occurring nature of HIV and substance use, studies that have examined efforts to improve ancillary health, mental health and social service provider's involvement in HIV medication adherence have not involved substance abuse counselors. This may be due to some studies requiring administration of complex standardized research instruments (Palmer, Saledo, Miller, Winiarski, & Arno, 2003; Stein et al., 2000). Although Klinkenberg and Sacks (2004) call for "consistency between primary treatment and ancillary services," and recognizing the need for substance abuse counseling, it is more of a call for physicians to obtain skills in mental health and substance abuse, not a call for mental health and substance abuse counselors to become skilled in supporting medication adherence (Klinkenberg & Sacks, 2004, p. S32, see also Loughlin et al., 2004).

RIME-EARS Stages of Change and Client Centered Counseling

The counseling method developed for the medication adherence is called the RIME-EARS intervention (Readiness, Initiation, Maintenance, Evaluation-Engage, Assess, Recommend, Support), which was developed as a best practice model for medical personnel (Linsk & Bonk, 2000; Linsk et al., 1998; Lubin et al., 1998). It is based upon a counseling model utilizing the transtheoretical stages of change model, which has been tested and found to contribute to counselors being better able to target appropriate interventions to support behavior change (Miller & Rollnick, 2002; Prochaska & DiClemente, 1998; Prochaska & DiClemente, 1982). Building on the trans-theoretical model, RIME-EARS recognizes that at different stages of behavior change clients and their counselors have different tasks. For example, in the RIME-EARS *readiness phase,* clients need help determining if they are ready to commence medication therapy; in the *initiation phase* clients may need support to solve problems associated with starting or changing the regimen; and in the *maintenance/evaluation* phase, the counselor may concentrate on monitoring and supporting progress and outcomes as well as resolving challenges associated with long term use of medication such as side effects. Client centered models of treatment have also been utilized to effect behavior change (Perlman, 1957; Reid & Epstein, 1972; Saybrook Graduate School and Research Center, 2002), and are also seen as both respectful to clients and encouraging of client empowerment.

Experiential Learning and Evaluation

Boud, Keough and Walker (cited in Merriam & Caffarella, 1999), reflecting on experiential learning for adults, indicate there are three stages to the process of learning from experience: "(1) returning and replaying the experience, (2) attending to the feelings that the experience provoked, and (3) reevaluating the experience" (p. 226). Patient simulation includes "a trained simulator who portrays relevant psychosocial and medical problems in a specific situation with a student who interacts with the client in conjunction with the course's main topics and training objectives" (Linsk & Tunney, 1997, p. 474), which has its roots in patient simulation/standardized patients used for training and evaluation in medical education (Barrows, 1993).

METHODS

Project Description

The program utilized a training platform, which included the following components: curricula slide presentations, trainer materials, videos, role-plays, and case simulation scripts and participant instructions. A training platform (J. Rosenfeld, personal communication, April 4, 2000) is a set of training tools assembled to inform an experienced trainer about a specific topic which can then be used to conduct an educational program. It is distinguished from a curriculum in that it is less proscriptive and allows the trainer to tailor the package to his or her own strengths based on the audience, and can be manualized and thus more easily disseminated. The platform was developed by the Midwest AIDS Training and Education Center (MATEC) in 1997 to train health professionals in HIV medication adherence based on the Midwest AIDS Training and Education Partners Adherence Initiative (See the AIDS Education and Training Resource, National Resource Center site for Training Platform Materials, 2006; Linsk & Bonk, 2000; Linsk, Lubin, Sherer, & Schechtman, 1998; Lubin, Linsk, Sherer, & Schechtman, 1998). The two primary MATEC trainers for this project had experience utilizing this platform with health providers since its inception. They were supervised by the principal investigators and provided oversight to the other trainers, client simulators, and observers.

Three substance abuse agencies agreed to participate and recruited their substance abuse counselors to a 1 1/2-day medication adherence training that consisted of both didactic and patient simulation components. Each participant received a folder containing slide presentations and supplementary materials. The full-day didactic training included information about HIV transmission, HAART, medication purposes, side effects, and drug interactions including Methadone. Client-centered adherence counseling based on "stages of change" was learned through slide presentations, handouts, and role-play demonstrations. In order to discuss medications with their clients, the SACs were presented a client-centered counseling approach to encourage counselors to listen to and support their client's informed decisions. The counseling also used an evidence-based practice model, the Transtheoretical Model of Change elaborated by Prochaska and DiClemente (1982, 1995) as one of its conceptual frameworks.

Counselors were encouraged to discuss medication adherence with their client by receiving information and skill based lectures and discussions about HIV medication and HIV medication adherence counseling, case based demonstrations as well as the use of video and experiential client-counselor simulations (Linsk & Tunney, 1997), which permitted participants to practice the skills. The client simulations were provided in a subsequent 1/2-day session in which counselors interviewed HIV-affected clients or other HIV knowledgeable individuals who served as training simulators. These simulations included a standardized case, which allowed participants to practice skills and receive feedback from the client simulators (in their client roles) as well as from training faculty who served as observers. These experiences provided the substance abuse counselors with opportunities to reflect on their practice through the prism of what they had learned about HIV medication and client centered counseling.

Training Evaluation

Instruments

The training was evaluated using a pre-test (before training), post-test (after training), and follow-up (six-months after training) design. The evaluation consisted of self-administered surveys that included questions about the counselors' practice activities, their comfort level discussing HIV medication and substance use with their clients and the client's physician, and the components of training they found most useful in their practice. The pre-test also obtained counselor and client demographic information, attitudes about HIV, substance abuse and medication; the post-test explored the extent to which practitioners expected to utilize practices they had learned; the follow-up-test assessed the degree to which various elements of the training had been implemented. Questions regarding attitudes or comfort levels used Likert scales. The questionnaire was based upon an earlier instrument used to assess case managers' prevention skills (Mitchell & Linsk, 2001), but was supplemented with additional questions related to treatment adherence and substance abuse. A unique identifier code was developed for each counselor each time they completed a survey in order to facilitate response matching while preserving the participants' confidentiality.

Analysis

Once collected, categorical and quantitative answers were entered into SPSS 12.0. Sample characteristics were summarized and variables of interest were analyzed using a primarily means comparisons and correlational strategy. Open-ended responses were compiled and manually coded to determine patterns of response, preferences and concerns. Answers to these questions that converged were categorized and coded to indicate the frequency of the counselors' responses (Aday, 1996; Miles & Huberman, 1994). Results of selected variables repeated or adapted in subsequent administrations of the survey (e.g., the post-test survey asked counselors which practices they expected to perform while follow-up ascertained which practices they had actually performed in the past three months) were compared. Data analysis included frequencies, proportions and other descriptive statistics. Paired sample t-tests were utilized to measure significance of mean differences and correlations were used to assess significance of rankings.

Project Sponsor and IRB

The project was undertaken by MATEC in collaboration with the Illinois Treatment Alternatives for Safe Communities (TASC) for the Chicago Practice Improvement Collaborative, a multi-agency consortium charged to improve intervention practices in substance abuse programs (Bass, Linsk, Mitchell, & Noel, 2006). The University Institutional Review Board (IRB) approved all aspects of the project. Counselors received continuing education credits for certification as an incentive to participate and complete all components of the program.

RESULTS

Demographics of Counselors and Their Clients

Forty-one counselors began the training and completed the first day's didactic presentation; 36 of these (87.8%) returned and completed the experiential practice simulation. All 36 subsequently completed the follow-up survey three months after training. Of these 36 participants only 29 had identifiers that could be matched and included in the analysis. Seventeen (58.6%) were female and twelve (41.4%) were male. The majority (58.6%) of participants were African American, six (20.7%) were Latino/a, five (17.2%) were White, and 1 (3.4%) was Asian, proportions that closely mirrored the ethnic/racial background they reported for their clients. The mean age of the counselors was 47.18 years, (range 26-76 years); over two-thirds of the counselors were over 40 years of age. Seventeen of the counselors (58.6%) had less than a college degree, 8 possessed a bachelor's degree and 4 had master's degrees. Sixteen counselors (55.1%) had over five years of experience in providing substance abuse counseling services. With the exception of three counselors, all had some form of counselor certification (e.g., Certified Substance Abuse Counselor).

The counselors varied regarding whether their clients had disclosed HIV positive status and use of HIV anti-retroviral medications. Nineteen of the counselors reported 182 clients had shared that they were HIV positive, indicating that nearly two-thirds of the counselors had seen at least one client reporting HIV. Seventeen (58.6%) of the counselors reported they had 148 clients who had shared with them they were taking HIV medications. See Table 1 for more details about demographics.

Survey Results

Counselors were asked questions at pre-test and post-test about their comfort levels before and after training with repeated case scenarios. Two open-ended sets of questions provided related feedback regarding how medication was most useful to them in their practice with HIV affected and non-affected clients; and counselors indicated strategies their clients and they would suggest to improve their substance-using client's medication adherence.

Comparative Analyses

Adherence Scenarios Comfort–Pre-Test and Post-Test Questions

In the pre-test survey five scenarios were presented to assess counselor comfort with addressing prevention and medication adherence issues

TABLE 1. Demographic Characteristics of Substance Abuse Counselors and Their Clients

Substance Abuse TX Participants Counselors (n = 29)		Counselor Estimate of Clients (n = 792)
Characteristics	Frequency	Frequency
Gender	41.4% Male	51.4% Male
	58.6% Female	39.0% Female*
Race/Ethnicity	58.6% African American	59.6% African American
	20.7% Hispanic	18.1% Hispanic
	17.2% White	13.35% White
	3.4% Asian	.8% Asian*
Education	58.6% < BA Degree	Clients share HIV Status n = 182
	37.9% ≥ BA Degree	Clients share HIV Med Status n = 148
Years SA Counseling	44.8% < 5 years	10 Counselors had no HIV clients
	55.2% > 5 years	11 Counselors had 1-3 HIV clients
		4 Counselors had 4+ HIV clients
		1 Counselor had 100 HIV clients

* These percentages are counselor estimations and did not add up to 100%.

with clients (Likert scaling 1 = very uncomfortable, 5 = very comfortable). Three case scenarios were repeated in the post-test to see if, after the adherence training, there were differences (compared to pre-test) in the counselors' comfort level related to (1) a client relapsing, (2) a client not taking medication, and (3) a counselor contacting the client's physician to advocate for medication. The advocacy scenario is presented below:

Client Advocacy with a Physician

Sam has been sober for two months, is complying with substance abuse treatment and building a healthy lifestyle. He now wants to attend to his HIV disease and begin HIV medication to maintain his health. His medical clinic informs him he must be sober at least six months before they will consider him for medication. He is concerned that his health will worsen if he does not start medication soon. He asks you, as his substance abuse counselor, to contact his physician about his adjustment in substance abuse treatment.

At baseline assessment, participants expressed the least amount of comfort in considering advocating for a client with a physician ($M = 3.97$). After training the post-test score for this item rose to 4.48, but this was not a statistically significant change. However, it was the only score among the post-test scenarios in which the mean score increased from the pre-test, which may reflect a trend. Scores of the Relapse and Medication Adherence scenarios decreased by a small amount in the post-test from 4.79 to 4.74 and 4.87 to 4.65 respectively. Notably, there were some statistical differences when comparing means of the three different scenarios at the pre and then the post-test. Significance for the paired scenarios was set at $p < .01$ to take into account the multiple responses being analyzed. At the pre-test the "Client Advocacy with a Physician" Scenario mean (3.97) when paired with the Relapse ($M = 4.79$) and the Medication Adherence Scenario ($M = 4.87$), SACs reported significantly less comfort contacting the physician ($p < .01$). In the post-test only the Relapse and Client Advocacy with a Physician means neared significant difference at $p < .03$ due to the increase in the post-test result for Client Advocacy with a Physician and the decrease of the Medical Adherence Scenario (see Table 2).

TABLE 2. Case Scenario–Comparison of Mean Responses

Scenario Pairs	Relapse Scenario	Medication Side Effects Scenario	Contact Physician Scenario	t-test/ Significance
Pre-test Pairs–Relapse, Medication, and Physician				
Pre-test–Pair 1				$t = -1.80$ $p = .083$
	4.79	4.90		
Relapse–Medication				
Pre-test–Pair 2				$t = 3.093,$
	4.79		3.97	
Relapse–Physician				$p = .004^*$
Pre-test–Pair 3				$t = 3.615,$
		4.87	3.97	
Medication–Physician				$p = .001^*$
Post-test Pairs–Relapse, Medication, and Physician				
Post-test Pair–Pair 1				$t = 1.45$
	4.74	4.65		
Relapse–Medication				$p = .162$
Post-test–Pair 2				$t = 2.31,$
	4.74		4.48	
Relapse–Physician				$p = .03$
Post-test–Pair 3				$t = 1.45,$
		4.65	4.48	
Medication–Physician				$p = .162$

*Statistically significant difference

Response to all three training scenarios were evaluated at two time points, that of pre and post-test. Pearson Correlation Coefficients were used to assess whether SACs who were comfortable in one of the scenarios also felt comfortable in another scenario. Significance for correlation coefficients of the scenarios was set at $p < .01$ to take into account the multiple responses being analyzed. Pre-test evaluation indicated that there was a very high coefficient of comfort in the scenarios for Relapse and Medication Adherence, $r = .778$ $p < .001$. The Physician Advocacy Scenario had extremely low level coefficients correlation with the other pre-test scenarios of Relapse ($r = .093$, $p = .631$) and Medication Adherence ($r = .180$, $p = .349$). At the post-test, the 23 participants responding had comfort levels in all the three scenarios that were correlated: Relapse and Medication Adherence had an even higher coefficient than at pre-test ($r = .813$, $p = .000$); Physician Advocacy had a high coefficient with both Relapse ($r = .589$, $p = .003$), and Medication Adherence ($r = .537$, $p = .008$).

Open-Ended Questions

Counselors responded to the open-ended questions below three months after they had completed the training. While it is not clear if the responses are based upon the training they received or from their prior experience, the SACs responses shared substance abuse counseling within the context of medication adherence and the health of their clients.

What Was Most Useful in Training?–Follow-up Survey

When asked at follow-up on an open-ended question what was "most useful" in the training for SACs for their HIV affected clients, about a third (10) of the counselors responded they valued understanding the medical effects of the medications. One counselor here noted drug interactions, how "using illicit drugs would affect HIV positive people responding to medication" was most useful.

Eight counselors felt the HIV medication information was most useful for them with their non-HIV affected clients as a means for prevention. Six counselors indicated that the information they received from training that certain medications should not be mixed with alcohol or drugs was the most useful information for their non-HIV affected clients.

What Strategies for HIV Medication Adherence SACs Developed?–
Follow-up Survey

At follow-up counselors shared ideas they and/or their clients developed to improve medication adherence. Some counselors told their clients about the health benefits of the medication to encourage their client's adherence. Strategies specific to substance abuse included encouragement to "maintain sobriety," "abstinence from illicit drugs," and "taking meds on time so as not to disrupt their methadone dosing." One counselor used an analogy that if the client didn't "take their methadone daily they may have problems–the same with adherence to taking their prescribed medication." Counselors also reported ideas such as the need for support groups and education. Medical personnel were acknowledged as playing an essential role in client's efforts to adhere, for example: "Reporting changes to the doctor," "Discussing medical issues with the MD." "Asking doctors and nurses to modify schedules to reduce side effects that impair performance." One counselor shared an agency oriented approach: their program rewarded clients with a pick-up of methadone, when clients adhere to their medication.

What Strategies for HIV Medication Adherence SACs Reported
Their Client Developed?–Follow-up Survey

A counselor posed that one of their clients shared the strategy of "not using drugs while on HIV meds" while another client's idea was they should "not substitute or share their medication with others." One client suggested to their counselor they needed to develop "habit forming rituals" for taking their medication. This idea might be based on patterns substance-using individuals may follow when they have to take their addictive illicit substances. Another idea shared was "giving them help for not adhering." The idea here may relate to "relapse prevention," that non-adherence should be expected, and therefore obtaining help for it should be planned.

Summary

The counselors' participation and their satisfaction comments indicate they were receptive to the medication portion of the training. The survey case examples reveal they were more comfortable discussing difficult issues with their clients than about advocating for their client with a physician. Their written comments provided insights into some of the recovery issues that clients might be facing and they provide a variety of ideas for ways to address medication adherence that reflect their substance-using clients' realities.

DISCUSSION AND IMPLICATIONS

While the findings indicated general satisfaction with the training and willingness to apply training in the practice settings, a number of issues emerged that provoke further research and education to improve practice. The findings suggest that substance abuse providers benefit from such training and may utilize knowledge and skills to improve their work with clients as well as health and service professionals; however, interaction with medical providers is seen as more difficult.

Communication with Clients and Physicians

The training evaluation revealed that some counselors had discomfort regarding communicating with medical professionals about medical issues and medications, not just HIV. Part of this may be a reluctance to cross professional boundaries and part may reflect the need for confidentiality in HIV and substance abuse treatment. However, with the complexity of treatment, substance abuse clients need to have support for their recovery, and part of that is making healthy decisions and maintaining healthy behavior. Substance abuse counselors, whose race/ethnicity in this study mirror their clients, may spend more time with their clients and know them better than a health professional. Their level of education also is closer to that of their clients than physicians and nurses; so if the counselor does not understand a health provider's instructions in a simulation or after training, it is also likely their client would also not comprehend either.

To improve practice, substance abuse counselors knowledgeable about HIV and medication adherence could enhance client understanding of what their client's doctor has told them, as well as communicate client concerns that health providers might overlook. This advocacy could result in better client decisions and improved medication adherence.

SACs Communicating About Recovery

Counselors also may be more likely to have greater cultural understanding of their client's background, not only because of racial/ethnic similarities, but also because some counselors may share a history of substance use recovery (Doyle, 1997). They also are more likely to have contact with this population. Cunningham (2000) reported on a study utilizing the National Longitudinal Alcohol Epidemiological Survey (NLAES, citing Grant) that 90.7% of respondents reporting having recovered from heroin use had "accessed treatment for addictions concerns at some point in their life" (p. 212). Methadone, an opioid substitute treatment, was utilized at the three clinics for this study. White and Kurtz (2005) view "medication-assisted recovery," as "medically monitored pharmacological adjuncts to support recovery from addiction" (p. 12), so those receiving methadone may be viewed as achieving recovery (White & Coon, 2003). Working with their clients on recovery and relapse prevention, substance abuse counselors might explain medication adherence so that their clients affected by substance use can understand it. A related implication for practice is that substance abuse counselors who have either experience and/or knowledge about the role of recovery in their clients' lives could be helpful in applying the concept of recovery in relationship to adherence. Understanding ways in which recovery and adherence apply to those with co-occurring substance use and HIV can assist both SACs and HIV health providers in improving their practice.

Substance Abuse Counselor's Counseling Competency in Pharmacotherapy

In addition to counseling techniques, substance abuse providers are trained in screening, assessment, referral and service coordination. The Substance Abuse and Mental Health Services Administration developed *Addiction Counseling Competencies,* a curriculum guide which calls on practitioners to be accepting of "pharmacotherapy" (Addiction Technology Transfer Centers [ATTC] National Curriculum Committee, 1998, pp. 17-18). It calls on counselors to be "knowledgeable [about] medical and pharmacological interventions" and to "understand the role medical problems and complications can play in…the treatment of addiction" (ATTC, p. 21). Therefore, while the substance abuse counselor is encouraged to utilize health resources, they are also called upon to understand the interaction between co-existing "medical and psychological disorders" (ATTC, p. 16). Batki and Selwyn (2000) recognize the role of substance abuse counselors in "models of integrated care" for those receiving HIV medication (p. 27). This implies that the development of integrated care models in which medical, mental health and substance abuse treatment are all provided in one or multiple settings, substance abuse counselors need to be included as an integral part of the health care team.

Limitations

Reliance on self-reported measures only did not allow for validation of the information received in terms of validity and reliability of attitude and motivation measures. Consequently, replications or additional applicable standardized measures need to be utilized in future studies. Some findings would have been strengthened had there been a follow-up with clients receiving these interventions. As a pilot, it was helpful to have some counselors involved who were not treating HIV affected clients, however the training would have more direct benefit to substance abuse counselors already working with HIV affected clients. Those counselors would have a more immediate need to know the information, and also to practice and apply the intervention model with clients for whom HIV medication adherence is an issue. Several cases were missing in this data set, because the name coding utilized did not effectively track the counselors through all three surveys. An assigned code for each participant might assist in better tracking of the surveys, but confidentiality safeguards would need to be addressed.

A drawback to this training was that some of the counselors' primary language was Spanish. An improvement would have made the training, surveys, and training materials available in Spanish. Despite these limitations this exploratory study does capture some of the experiences of the learners, both within the training and at follow-up and sets the stage for future research.

CONCLUSION

Future training studies might consider evaluating the ways and the extent to which agencies participating in a "knowledge application study" incorporate and utilize any of the practices learned by staff (Ingersoll & Heckman, 2005). Training programs may encourage more discussions about medication effects in the simulations, or on-site in "real" counseling settings. Another possibility would be cross-training with health professionals and substance abuse counselors, so both groups have an opportunity to discuss the relationship between the health and recovery of co-occurring clients (Batki & Selwyn, 2002).

This sample of SACs tended to be similar to their clients in ethnic background, and educational level. These similarities along with the greater amount of contact clients have with their SACs than with their physician make it possible for those SACs trained in HIV medication adherence to provide additional support to clients facing decisions or needing support regarding HAART regiments and other medical regimens. Some of the lower comfort level of the SACs in the physician case scenario may be explained by confidentiality requirements, or from education, cultural and professional barriers. However, these barriers need to be overcome if better communication is to occur, thereby offering the prospect of improved health for persons living with HIV and co-occurring substance use.

ACKNOWLEDGMENTS

This study was part of the *HIV Adherence Training for Substance Abuse Counselors: A Knowledge Application Replication Project.* The Chicago Practice Improvement Collaborative provided support, administered by the Illinois Treatment Alternatives for Safe Communities (TASC) and funded by the Center for Substance Abuse Treatment (CSAT), Grant No. 1 UD1 TI12900-03. Additional support was provided by the Midwest AIDS Training and Education Center (Health Resources and Services Administration Grant No. 6 H4AH0062-05-01) and the Great Lakes Addictions Technology Transfer Center (Substance and Mental Health Services Administration Grant Number 6UD1TI13593-04-1). The authors acknowledge the helpful support, and involvement of the administration, and the participation and ideas shared by the staff of Cornell Interventions Inc, El Rincon Community Clinic, and Substance Abuse Services Inc, Chicago, IL. Special thanks are given to the staff of Midwest AIDS Training and Education Center and the Great Lakes Addictions Technology Transfer Center. Eric Noel, Elyse Nowak, Bethsheba Johnson, and Veronica Montgomery expertly provided this training and made the materials relevant to the counselors. Anthony Oltean assisted with data analysis. The authors also wish to express our gratitude to Arthur Lurigio, Loyola University and Treatment Alternatives to Safe Communities (TASC) Beth Epstein, PIC Coordinator, Melody Heaps and Pamela Rodriguez, Chicago Practice Improvement Collaborative at TASC, who provided administrative leadership, support and direction necessary to carry out this program.

REFERENCES

Aday, L. A. (1996). *Designing and conducting health surveys: Second edition.* San Francisco: Jossey-Bass, A Wiley Company.

Addiction Technology Transfer Centers (ATTC), National Curriculum Committee (1998). Addiction counseling competencies: The knowledge, skills, and attitudes of professional practice: Technical assistance publication series 21. Substance Abuse

156   *HIV TREATMENT ADHERENCE*

and Mental Health Services Administration, Rockwall II, 5600 Fishers Lane, Rockville, MD, DHHS Publication No. [SMA] 98-3171.

AIDS Education and Training Center, National Resource Center. (2006). *Training Platform Materials.* Retrieved on September 4, 2006 at http://www.aidsetc.org/aidsetc?page=et-00-01

Bamberger, J. D., Unick, J., Klein, P., Fraser, M., Chesney, M., & Katz, M. H. (2000). Helping urban poor stay with antiretroviral HIV drug therapy. *American Journal of Public Health, 90* (5), 699-701.

Bangsberg, D. R., Hecht, F. M., Charlebois, E. D., Zolopa, A. R., Holodniy, M., Sheiner, L. et al. (2000). Adherence to protease inhibitors, HIV-01 viral load and development of drug resistance in an indigent population. *AIDS, 14,* 357-366.

Bangsberg, D., Tulsky, J., Hecht, F., & Moss, A. (1997). Protease inhibitors in the homeless. *Journal of the American Medical Association, 287,* 63-65.

Barrows, H. (1993). An overview of the uses of standardized patients for teaching and evaluating clinical skills. *Academic Medicine, 68,* 443-453.

Barthwell, A. G. (1997). Substance use and the puzzle of adherence. *Focus: A guide to AIDS research and counseling, 12,* 1-3.

Bass, M., Linsk, N., Mitchell, C., & Noel, E. (2006 February). *Adherence counseling training: HIV adherence training for substance abuse counselors: A knowledge application replication: Final report prepared for the Chicago Practice Improvement Collaborative and Treatment Alternative for Safe Communities.* Midwest AIDS Training and Education Center, Chicago.

Batki, S. L., & Selwyn, P. A. (2002). *Substance abuse treatment for persons with HIV/AIDS: Treatment improvement protocol (TIP) series: 37.* U.S. Department of Health and Human Services, Public Health Service, Substance Abuse and Mental Health Services Administration, Center for Substance Abuse Treatment, Rockwall II, 5600 Fishers Lane, Rockville, MD 20857.

Carpenter, C. J., Cooper, D. A., Fischl, M. A., Gatell, J. M., Gazzard, B. G., Hammer, S. M. et al. (2000). Antiretroviral therapy in adults: Updated recommendations of the International AIDS Society–USA Panel. *Journal of the American Medical Association, 283* (3), 381-391.

Centers for Disease Control and Prevention. (1998). *HIV, TB & infectious diseases: The alcohol and other drug use connection: A practical approach to linking clients to treatment: Participant guide.* Center for Substance Abuse Treatment, Substance Abuse and Mental Health Services Administration, Rockville, MD, DHHS publication no. (SMA) 98-3202, 107 p.

Centers for Disease Control and Prevention. (2002). *Drug-associated HIV transmission continues in the United States.* Centers for Disease Control. Retrieved on February 13, 2006 at http://www.cdc.gov/hiv/pubs/facts/idu.htm.

Chaison, R. E., Keruly, J. C., & Moore, R. D. (1995). Race, sex, drug use and progression of HIV. *New England Journal of Medicine, 333,* 751-756.

Chesney, M. A. (2000). Factors affecting adherence to antiretroviral therapy. *Clinical Infectious Diseases.* (Suppl.2): S171-176.

Cunningham, C. O., & Selwyn, P. A. (2005). HIV-related medical complications and treatment. In J. H. Lowinson, P. Ruiz, R. B. Millman, & J. G. Langrod (Eds.), *Substance abuse: A comprehensive* textbook (4th ed., pp. 922-987). Lippincott, Williams, & Wilkins: Philadelphia.

Cunningham, J. A. (2000). Remissions from drug dependence: Is treatment a prerequisite? *Drug and Alcohol Dependence, 59,* 211-213.

DiClemente, C., Prochaska, J., Velicer, W., Fairhurst, S., Rossi, J., & Valasquez, M. (1991). The process of smoking cessation: An analysis of precontemplation, contemplation, and preparation stages of change. *Journal of Consulting and Clinical Psychology, 59,* 295-304.

Doyle, K. (1997). Substance abuse counselors in recovery: Implications for the ethical issues of dual relationships. *Journal of Counseling and Development, 75,* 428-432.

Frank, L., & Miramontes, H. (1999). AIDS Education and Training Center adherence curriculum. HIV InSite. University of California at San Francisc, Center for HIV Information. Retrieved on July 27, 2006 at http://hivinsite.org/InSite?page=md-rr-04.

Health Resources and Human Services Administration (2005, January). HRSA fact sheets: Substance Abuse and HIV. Author. Retrieved on December 19, 2005 at http://hab.hrsa.gov/history/fact2005/substance_abuse_and_hivaids.htm.

Ingersoll, K. S., & Heckman, C. J. (2005). Patient-Clinician relationships and treatment system effects on HIV medication adherence. *AIDS and Behavior, 9* (1), 89-101.

Johnson, M. O., Catz, S. L., Remien, R. H., Rotheram-Borus, M. J., Morini, S. F., Charlebois, E. et al. (2003). Theory-guided, empirically supported avenues for intervention on HIV medication on HIV medication non-adherence: Finding from the Healthy Living Project. *AIDS Patient Care and STDs, 17* (12), 645-656.

Klinkenberg, W. D., & Sacks, S. (2004). Mental disorders and drug abuse in persons living with HIV/AIDS. *AIDS Care, 16*(Suppl. 1), S22-S42.

Linsk, N. L., & Bonk, N. (2000). Adherence to Treatment as Social Work Challenges. In V. Lynch (Ed.), *HIV/AIDS at the year 2000: A sourcebook for social workers.* Boston: Allyn & Bacon, 211-227.

Linsk, N. L., Lubin, B., Sherer, R., & Schechtman, B. A. (1998). *The MATEC adherence initiative, Midwest AIDS Training and Education partners.* Midwest AIDS Training Center, Chicago, IL.

Linsk, N. L., & Tunney, K. (1997). Learning to care: Use of practice simulation to train health social workers. *Journal of Social Work Education, 33*(3), 473-489.

Loughlin, A., Metsch, L., Gardner, L., Anderson-Mahoney, P., Barrigan, M., & Strathdee, S. (2004). Provider barriers to prescribing HAART to medically-eligible HIV-infected drug users. *AIDS Care, 16*(4), 485-500.

Lubin, B., Linsk, N., Sherer, R., & Schechtman, B. (1998). *The Midwest AIDS Training and Education Partners (MATEP) adherence initiative: Rationale and goals* [abstract no. 32381]. XII International AIDS Conference, Geneva, Switzerland.

Lucas, G. M., Gebo, K. A., Chaisson, R. E., & Moore, R. D. (2002). Longitudinal assessment of the effects of drug and alcohol on HIV-1 treatment outcomes in an urban clinic. *AIDS 16* (5), 767-774.

Merriam, S. B., & Caffarella, R. S. (1999). *Learning in adulthood: A comprehensive guide* (2nd ed.). San Francisco: Josey-Bass Publishers.

Miles, M. B., & Huberman, A. M. (1994). *Qualitative data analysis: An expanded sourcebook* (2nd edition). Thousand Oaks, CA: Sage.

Miller, W. R., & Rollnick, S.(2002). *Motivational interviewing: Preparing people for change.* New York, NY: Guilford Press.

Mitchell, C. G., & Linsk, N. (2001). Prevention for positives: Challenges and opportunities for integrating secondary prevention into HIV case management. *AIDS Education and Prevention, 13*, 393-402.

Newcomer, K. E. (1994). Using statistics appropriately. In J. S. Wholey, H. P. Hatry, & K. E. Newcomer (Eds.), *Handbook of Practical Program Evaluation*. San Francisco: Josey-Bass Publishers.

Palmer, N. B., Salcedo, J., Miller, A. L., Winiarske, M., & Arno, P. (2003). Psychiatric and social barriers to HIV medication adherence in a triply diagnosed methadone population. *AIDS Patient Care and STDs, 17* (12), 635-644.

Paterson, D., Swindells, S., Mohr, J., Brester, M., Vergis, E., Squier, C. et al. (1999). How much adherence is enough? A prospective study of adherence to protease inhibitor therapy using MEMS caps. *6th Conference on Retroviruses and Opportunistic Infections*. Chicago, Abstract #92.

Patterson, D. L., Swindells, S., Mohr, J., Brester, M., Vergis, E. N., Squier, C. et al. (2000). Adherence to protease inhibitor therapy and outcomes in patients with HIV infection. *Annals of Internal Medicine, 133* (1), 21-30.

Perlman, H. H. (1957). *Social Casework: A problem-solving approach*. Chicago, IL: The University of Chicago Press.

Prochaska, J. O., & DiClementi, C. C. (1998). Transtheoretical therapy: Toward a more integrated model of change. *Psychotherapy Theory, Research, and Practice, 19*, 276-288.

Prochaska, J. O., & DiClemente, C. C. (1982). Transtheoretical therapy: Toward a more integrated model of change. *Psychotherapy Theory, Research and Practice, 19* (3), 276-288.

Reid, W., & Epstein, L. (1972). *Task-centered casework*. New York, NY: Columbia University Press.

Saybrook Graduate School and Research Center (2002, July). Carl Rogers Symposium 2002: *Honoring 100 years of Carl R. Rogers: His life, our work, a global vision*. Presented by the University of California, San Diego at LaJolla, CA. Retrieved on November 29, 2005 at http://www.saybrook.edu/crr/

Sherer, R. (1998). Adherence and antiretroviral therapy in injection drug users. *Journal of the American Medical Association, 280* (6), 567-568.

Sollitto, S., Mehlman, M., Youngner, S., & Lederman, M. M. (2001). Should physicians withhold highly active antiretroviral therapies from HIV-AIDS patients who are thought to be poorly adherent to treatment? *AIDS 15*, 153-159.

Stein, M. D., Urdaneta, M. E., Clarke, J., Maksad, J., Sobota, M., Hanna, L. et al. (2000). Use of antiretroviral therapies by HIV-infected persons receiving methadone maintenance. *Journal of Addictive Diseases, 19*, 85-94

Ware, N. C., Wyatt, M. A., & Tugenberg, T. (2005). Adherence, stereotyping and unequal HIV treatment for active users of illegal drugs. *Social Science & Medicine, 61*, 565-576.

White, W., & Kurtz, E. (2005). *The varieties of recovery experience: A primer for addiction treatment professionals and recovery advocates*. Chicago, IL: Great Lakes Addiction Technology Transfer Center. Retrieved on November 16, 2005 at http://www.unhooked.com/discussion/VarietiesofRecoveryExperiencefinal 10-3-2005.pdf.

White, W. L., & Coon, B. F. (2003, October). Methadone and the anti-medication bias in addiction treatment. *Counselor, The Magazine for Addiction Professionals, 4*(5), 58-63. Retrieved on July 28, 2006 at http://www.counselormagazine.com/pfv.asp?aid = oct03Methadone.htm.

doi:10.1300/J187v06n01_09

More Than Drugs:
Voices of HIV-Seropositive Individuals with a History of Substance Use Reveal a Range of Adherence Factors

Dorie J. Gilbert, PhD, LMSW
Elizabeth Abel, PhD, RNC-FNP, FAANP
Nancy Francisco Stewart, PhD, ACSW
Margarita Zilberman, BA

Dorie J. Gilbert, PhD, LMSW, is Associate Professor, School of Social Work, The University of Texas at Austin, and Visiting Professor, Center for AIDS Prevention Studies, University of California at San Francisco.

Elizabeth Abel, PhD, RNC-FNP, FAANP, is Retired Associate Professor and Chair-Division of Family and Public Health Nursing, School of Nursing, The University of Texas at Austin.

Nancy Francisco Stewart, PhD, ACSW, is Assistant Professor, Department of Sociology and Social Work at Jacksonville State University, Jacksonville, AL.

Margarita Zilberman, BA, is a graduate research assistant, School of Social Work, The University of Texas at Austin and former HIV test counselor and prevention educator at the Geffen Testing Center at Gay Men's Health Crisis (GMHC) in New York City.

Address correspondence to: Dr. Dorie Gilbert, School of Social Work, University of Texas at Austin, 1 University Station D 3500, Austin, TX 78712 (E-mail: dgm@mail.utexas.edu).

The authors would like to thank the individuals who participated in the study.

This project was funded by the National Institute of Drug Abuse Pilot Study (1R24DA 13579-01A1).

[Haworth co-indexing entry note]: "More Than Drugs: Voices of HIV-Seropositive Individuals with a History of Substance Use Reveal a Range of Adherence Factors." Gilbert, Dorie J. et al. Co-published simultaneously in *the Journal of HIV/AIDS & Social Services* (The Haworth Press, Inc.) Vol. 6, No. 1/2, 2007, pp. 161-179; and: *HIV Treatment Adherence: Challenges for Social Services* (ed: Lana Sue Ka'opua and Nathan L. Linsk) The Haworth Press, Inc., 2007, pp. 161-179. Single or multiple copies of this article are available for a fee from The Haworth Document Delivery Service [1-800-HAWORTH, 9:00 a.m. - 5:00 p.m. (EST). E-mail address: docdelivery@haworthpress.com].

Available online at http://jhaso.haworthpress.com
doi: 10.1300/J187v06n01_10

SUMMARY. This study sought to uncover the prevalence of continued drug use and statements about everyday adherence decision-making from a community sample of HIV-seropositive individuals with a history of substance use and also enrolled in antiretroviral therapy (ART) for at least six months. Ninety participants attended one of three focus groups and, collectively, generated 100 statements describing their day-to-day motivations and barriers to HIV-medical adherence. In addition, participants' self-reported substance use revealed that just under 40% ($n = 33$) were juggling substance use and their HIV medication regimens within the past 30 days. The statements reveal varied and complex adherence factors, which included relatively more non-drug-related than drug-related factors. Further, participants non-drug-related statements covered a broad range of reasons related to adherence that tended to fall into the same major categories as those found across other subgroups: system, disease management, patient-provider relationship, and individual factors. The authors discuss the need for providers to consider the breath and complexity of adherence factors that impact readiness to initiate and adhere to ART for this population. doi:10.1300/J187v06n01_10
[Article copies available for a fee from The Haworth Document Delivery Service: 1-800-HAWORTH. E-mail address: <docdelivery@haworthpress.com> Website: <http:// www.HaworthPress.com> © 2007 by The Haworth Press, Inc. All rights reserved.]

KEYWORDS. HIV, AIDS, adherence, substance use, stigma

BACKGROUND

Adherence to antiretroviral therapy (ART) is crucial for its effectiveness in prolonging the lives of individuals with HIV disease; and despite some discussion to the contrary, with proper adherence, the effectiveness of ART should be the same across all HIV risk groups, including drug using populations (Vlahov & Celentano, 2006). Yet, compared to other HIV-seropositive groups, persons living with HIV who also have a history of substance use are less likely to be receiving ART. Rates of access may be low because some among this group choose not to be engaged in available services; others are part of "hidden populations" outside the reach of medical and social services. Further, people with substance use disorders, both past and current, contend with a great deal of societal stigma and stereotyping, which can bias medical and social service providers' attitudes towards them.

Thus, another reason for this group's lack of access to services is providers' perceptions of them as "poor" candidates for ART regimens based on assumptions of low adherence capabilities (Bangsberg et al., 2001; Bassetti, Battegay, & Surrer, 1999; Celentano et al., 1998; Clarke et al., 2003; Turner et al., 2001). Even when they do have access, people living with HIV and substance use are reported to have comparatively poor outcomes with adherence and retention in ART therapy (Arnsten et al., 2002; Gebo, Keruly, & Moore, 2003; Ingersoll, 2004; Johnson et al., 2006; Power et al., 2003; Tucker, Burnam, Sherbourne, Kung, & Gifford, 2003). This is of great concern because inconsistent use of ART medications and continued drug use may lead to rapid progression of HIV disease, reduced life expectancy, and, potentially, to the development and transmission of resistant strains of HIV (Adam, Maticka-Tyndale, & Cohen, 2003; Bangsberg, Hecht, & Charlebois, 2000; Sorensen et al., 1998). These concerns underscore the need to (1) explore the extent to which drug use co-occurs with ART; and, (2) develop a comprehensive understanding of facilitators and barriers to adherence for this population.

When we look at adherence research across the general population of HIV-seropositive individuals, factors associated with ART adherence have tended to fall within four categories: systemic factors, individual factors, disease management, and patient-provider relationship (Ickovics & Meade, 2002). Systemic factors include the extent to which individuals have access to insurance, medical and social services (Chesney et al., 2000). Patient-provider relationship factors impacting adherence include the provider's beliefs about the patient (Gifford et al., 2000), the patient's knowledge and understanding of the regimen (Stone, Hogan & Schuman, 2001), and quality of communication with the physician/ provider (Kremer & Ironson, 2006).

Disease management and treatment factors shown to be associated with non-adherence to ART are severity of HIV symptoms, complexity of the treatment regimen, and medication side effects (Uldall, Palmer, Whetten, & Mellins, 2004). Side effects commonly cited as adherence barriers include anemia, neuropathy, hyperglycemia, diarrhea, nausea, fatigue, headaches and fat redistribution (Montessori, Press, Harris, Akagi, & Montaner, 2004). Another common disease management factor is forgetting to take a pill (Barfod, Sorensen, Nielsen, Rodkjaer, & Obel, 2006), especially given complicated medication schedules that often require taking multiple pills several times a day (da Silveira,

Drachler, Leite, & Pinheiro, 2003). Individual factors, including mental health disorders (Arnsten et al., 2002; Mellins, Kang, Leu, Havens, & Chesney, 2003; Tucker et al., 2003; Read, Mijch, & Fairley, 2003), social support (Malcolm, Ng, Rosen, & Stone, 2003; Power et al., 2003), and attitudes about ART (Johnson et al., 2003) have also been found to influence adherence outcomes.

Among people living with HIV and past or current substance use disorders, commonly cited non-adherence factors are drug use and unstable lifestyles (Gebo et al., 2003; Golin et al., 2002; Haubrich et al., 1999; Lucas, Cheever, Chaisson, & Moore, 2001; Vlahov & Celentano, 2006). Studies have found that substance users may become non-adherent because of concern about the interaction between drugs and ART (Reback, Larkins, & Shoptaw, 2003); and recovering drug users have also expressed concern about ingesting medication and may associate the difficulties of taking the medication with the constraints of drug abuse (Oggins, 2003). Among injected drug users (IDUs) specifically, the most frequently cited reasons for discontinuing ART is becoming incarcerated (Altice, Mostashari, & Friedland, 2001), but more recently Kerr et al. (2005) found side effects as well as incarceration to be crucial barriers. In general, studies on suboptimal adherence for certain subgroups help us tailor interventions, but they may also unintentionally limit our understanding of the broader adherence dynamics among this subgroup (Ware, Wyatt, & Tugenberg, 2005). Recent descriptive studies have helped to disentangle the assumptions about substance users by distinguishing between active and non-active substance use as well as non-drug-related factors that influence adherence outcomes (Martini et al., 2004; Ware et al.). This paper further explores the intricate realities of ART adherence, specifically among HIV-seropositive individuals identifying themselves as having a *history* of substance misuse.

This study sought to uncover (1) the prevalence of continued drug use and (2) statements about everyday adherence decision-making from a community sample of HIV-seropositive individuals with a history of substance use disorders and who were also enrolled in ART for at least six months. The focus groups were part of a larger pilot study to develop an evaluative tool to assess readiness to initiate ART for this population. As an initial step, we needed to assess the range of cognitive and behavioral processes they may experience while attempting to maintain ART adherence; processes which likely exist on a continuum of psychosocial factors that facilitate or inhibit change. Toward that aim, we set out to elicit a comprehensive list of adherence factors; essentially, we wanted to hear–directly from those affected–the full range of their reasons for adhering or not.

METHODOLOGY

This exploratory study employed focus groups guided by the concept mapping methodology (Trochim, 1989). Concept mapping organizes complex ideas generated by participants into conceptual frameworks, and entails two phases: (1) qualitative elicitation research to generate ideas and statements from participants on the research question and, (2) subsequent quantitative analyses of participants' responses. This paper focuses on the *first* phase of this methodology, the qualitative elicitation research, because of its utility in allowing the researchers to capture the spontaneous voice of the participants. We were specifically interested in generating comments from the participants that provided an exhaustive list of reasons, both pros and cons, for adhering *or not* on a day-to-day basis.

Participants. Focus group participants were 90 HIV-positive adults in an urban metropolitan area in the southern United States who had a history of substance use. Forty-seven percent were African American/ Black, 24% Hispanic/Latino, 26% White, and 1% Asian American. Ages ranged from 18 to 50; and the majority (83%) was between 30 to 60 years of age. Seventy-three percent were male, 23% female, and 4% transgender.

Procedure. The research protocol was evaluated and approved by the lead authors' university institutional review board. Fliers describing the study were posted in several community-based organizations providing substance abuse services and/or HIV-related medical and social ser-vices. The fliers instructed potential participants in the procedures for volunteering for the study. Qualifications for the study included being over age 18, having a history of substance use, and active involvement with an HIV medication regimen for at least the past 6 months. Follow-ing informed consent procedures and before the focus groups, partici-pants completed a brief questionnaire which addressed the following areas: subject demographics; support group involvement; HIV, AIDS and Hepatitis C (HCV) status; and self-reported past and current sub-stance use.

The purpose of the focus groups was to bring the participants together to brainstorm a thorough list of statements about their reasons for taking or not taking HIV meds. As is used in concept mapping, the brainstorming was guided by a prompt; in this case we used the following open-ended prompt:

> *When I am deciding about taking my HIV medications, I think about . . .*

Participants were asked to generate responses in the form of phrases that described thoughts, emotions and behaviors that went into their daily decision-making about their medical regimens. Three focus groups, conducted over one week, resulted in an exhaustive list of reasons associated with taking or not taking HIV meds as reported by the participants. Ninety participants took part in the brainstorming focus groups. Of this 90 participants, 87 individuals completed demographic sheets.

Data Analysis. Data collected from the demographic questionnaires were analyzed descriptively to provide a demographic profile of the study participants; data on prevalence and type of drug use were analyzed by percentage and frequency distributions. After the focus groups, researchers transcribed the statements; duplicate statements made by more than one person were combined. After this reductive strategy, 100 statements remained. Because we were interested in elucidating as many different categories of reasons stated by participants, the statements were labeled in broad themes representing the range of responses of what participants said about motivators and barriers. Statements are presented here according to themes based first on two distinguishing categories, drug-related and non-drug-related factors. We then further analyzed the non-drug-related factors into categories reflecting the themes previously identified in the general population of HIV-seropositive individuals.

FINDINGS

Demographics, HIV, AIDS, and HCV Status

Participants were primarily male (73%) and a relatively older group; only 15 individuals (17%) were under 30 years of age. On average, participants had 5 years of experience with taking ART, and the mean number of years for being diagnosed with HIV was eight. Thirty-two of the 87 participants (37%) self-identified as having HCV co-infection; however, only a quarter of those individuals were receiving HCV treatment.

Forty-four percent (*n* = 39) of the participants were members of sub-stance abuse treatment support groups; another 18% (*n* = 15) were members of HIV-services support groups. Fifty-four of the 87 individu-als (62%) self-identified as having a history of injected drug use.

Prevalence of Current Drug Use

Nearly 50% (*n* = 43) of participants self-reported drug and/or alcohol use in the past six months; 33 participants reported use in the past 30 days. Of those using in the past 30 days, the most commonly used substances were alcohol (53%), marijuana (34%), crack-cocaine (29%), cocaine (27%), and injected drugs (24%). In many instances, poly-drug use (e.g., crack cocaine, marijuana, and alcohol) was characteristic. Over-all, just under 40% (*n* = 33) were juggling substance use and their HIV medication regimens within the past 30 days.

Focus Group Responses

Once presented with the research prompt, participants across all three focus groups spontaneously contributed a range of adherence factors. As a preliminary step, we categorized their reasons, first in terms of being drug- or non-drug-related. For drug-related factors, we included any statement referencing drug use or recovery. Within the non-drug-related factors we further explored sub-topics based on the participants' responses and the adherence themes emerging from previous research on the general population of seropositive individuals.

Drug-Related Factors

Of the 100 statements, participants generated a total of 13 responses reflecting substance use or recovery themes. The statements revealed their struggle with continued substance use. However, one participant shared that a daily reminder of himself as a "person in recovery" is a strong motivator to adhere successfully, stating with emphasis that:

> *About being a recovering person: a recovering addict takes the meds "as prescribed."*

Others participants revealed a more difficult struggle with decisions about continued drug use versus taking the medications, specifically around using marijuana to cope with side effects, but also expressed concerns about the legality of this:

> *If I am going to have all these side effects, I might as well smoke a joint.*
>
> *The fact that my using marijuana is illegal, even though it helps the side effects.*

One participant revealed how the HIV medications themselves interact with drug use:

> *Sustiva gives me a buzz and makes me want to use drugs more.*

Several statements highlight the ways in which participants were weighing the continued drug use against adherence, revealing both questions and concerns about the impact of drug use:

> *If I take them and then go on to use drugs, how is it going to affect the potency?*
>
> *The impact of using drugs on the HIV medication.*
>
> *They have to find a new regimen for my HIV meds if I stop the meds because I am using drugs.*
>
> *Doing drugs affects the medicine.*

Other drug-related statements reflected choosing drug use as a coping mechanism to mask the reality of their HIV disease, but also in response to a lack of social support, specifically from family:

> *The HIV meds take away the denial. To deal with the denial, I use drugs.*
>
> *If I am taking drugs I do not think about taking medicine.*
>
> *If my family doesn't care about me, I am going to use drugs.*
>
> *When I use drugs, I don't care about the HIV meds.*

A final statement revealed the struggle of disclosure of one's substance abuse to providers, specifically the physician:

> *Am I going to tell my doctor about my substance abuse?*

Overall, there were relatively few drug-related statements presented by the participants across the three focus groups.

Focus Group Responses: Non-Drug-Related Factors

The vast majority of psychological and behavioral struggles mentioned by participants did not specifically reference drugs or drug use. Non-drug-related statements are presented in thematic categories based on how we saw participants' responses fitting with the existing general adherence literature.

System-Level Factors

Participants identified system-level facilitators, including access and service provision factors, in the following statements:

> *There are great support groups.*
> *How lucky I am to live in America where I can get my meds.*
> *Services are good, access to medications, affordable.*

Systemic barriers identified included lack of access to medications while incarcerated, unstable housing, and Medicaid policies:

> *In the penitentiary, they do not have enough meds.*
> *Hard to adhere to my meds if I am living on the streets.*
> *Temporary living arrangements and people knowing my personal business.*
> *I worry about losing my benefits if I get too healthy.*

In addition to stigma, participants identified not only inadvertent disclosure of their status but also fear of violence as a barrier to taking medication, as indicated in the following statements:

> *Stigma.*
> *Is someone going to ask me why I'm taking the meds?*
> *I am afraid of physical retaliation if people know about my status.*

Individual Factors

Individual factors such as social support, attitudes about the disease, and mental health concerns such as depression were also identified.

Statements reflected observations similar to other research, in that participants' positive attitude, life purpose, and social support were indicated as motivating factors:

Positive Attitude and Acceptance

> *I don't have to let the disease beat me.*
> *A sense of empowerment; you control your own destiny .*
> *About how a positive attitude impacts how you respond to HIV.*
> *That I have accepted that I am sick.*
> *I re-frame it as a reward rather than a burden.*

Life purpose:

> *I think about God, being spiritual.*
> *I can continue to take care of my kids.*
> *Keeping a fulltime job.*

Social support and the lack thereof were identified as pros and cons, respectively:

> *The support I get from my family.*
> *The lack of support from my family.*
> *About friends and family who do not support me taking my meds.*

Patient-Provider Factors

Statements related to the patient-physician relationship also emerged, and all point to barriers based on accessibility concerns, poor communication, and lack of trust:

> *That I will run out of medication and not be able to track down the doctor.*
> *Do I really need the dosage that the doctor has prescribed?*
> *Lack of trust when the doctor terminates medications that are working.*
> *Am I getting a placebo?*

That the doctor tries out medications without testing its impact before.

My doctor is a quack.

Disease and Treatment Management

The majority of the statements fell into the category of disease and treatment management, and included statements about what helped participants in their struggles to effectively manage their regimen, such as routine, information, and wanting to live:

The need for the routine in order to stay healthy

If I won't do it religiously, why do it?

The need to educate myself about my illness.

I take them to avoid going in to the hospital.

I will stay undetected

The scariness of dying.

If I can just hang around until they make better drugs.

Barriers to adherence which related to disease management were depression, the burden of too many pills, fears and questions about the medications, and mistrust

I get depressed thinking about dying.

pills are a constant reminder of how I got the disease.

I think about all the pills, even the ones that are not for HIV but for depression, etc.

Would I rather live for ten years being happy without the meds or 30 more years being sick with the meds?

How long will it take before I become resistant to the medications?

I am tired of taking meds.

Not worth it because of no progress.

A lack of trust of the medication.

Am I taking the right regimen?

If the government wasn't truthful about HIV/AIDS, can I trust that there is not a cure that we are not given because the drug companies are making so much money.

That nobody is paying attention to how the meds cause different side effects for different ethnic groups.

As with other research, concerns, primarily in the form of questions, were raised about side effects, toxicity and drug resistance:

I am frightened because I do not know what the side affects will be.
Will the meds make me sicker than the HIV?
What damage are the meds doing to my body?
Is the medication mutating, "changing" the virus?
About the fact that the meds are so toxic.
If I get OFF the meds, will I also get side effects?
It messes with the sex drive.
I don't want to take it because of nightmares and hallucinations.

Several concerns raised were specific to those with HIV/HCV co-infection, and they reveal participants' questions and frustrations in their adherence struggles:

How do the Hepatitis C and HIV drugs interact?
What impact are the meds having on my Hepatitis C?
They are going to come out with a cure for HIV but not Hepatitis C.
That they are going to pull the same shit with Hepatitis C.

DISCUSSION

Overall, the findings point to a population that is actively grappling with adherence, and, for some, juggling adherence and substance use. Among those self-reporting drug and/or alcohol use in the past 30 days, the most commonly used substance was alcohol, which was used alone or with another drug by more than 50% of those reporting use in past 30 days. Alcohol use alone has been shown to have a negative association with self-reported adherence (Cook et al., 2001; Wagner et al., 2001), and the same goes for alcohol and drug use together. In a prospective cohort study ($n = 140$) of long-term adherence to HIV medications, Golin et al. (2002) found that those actively using drugs and those drinking alcohol adhered less well than non-users and non-drinkers. In our sample, marijuana use was the second most commonly used drug, followed by crack-cocaine and cocaine, but it is unclear if these drugs impact adherence equally. Tucker et al. (2003) found that cocaine and crack-cocaine as well as the use of sedatives, amphetamines, or marijuana in the past month were linked to non-adherence to ART. However, in another study, the use of marijuana alone was not associated with subjects (*n* = 252) self-reported adherence to antiretroviral therapy (Prentiss, Balmas, Power, & Israelski, 2002). Further, in their interviews with active drug users, Ware et al. (2005) found that drug users reported being able to take HIV medications when using cocaine, heroin, or marijuana, but not when smoking crack. Particularly interesting was our finding that current IDU was relatively uncommon in our sample. Considering that 54% of the 87 participants identified as having a history of IDU (mostly over 1-2 years), very few (*n* = 7) reported use of injected drugs in the past month; thus, the majority of IDUs were non-active users, which has been associated with better adherence outcomes (Aloisi et al., 2002). In addition, very few of our participants indicated use of inhalants or lub drugs, such as MDMA (ecstasy), inhalant nitrates, ketamine, or hallucinogens; however, these drugs have also been shown to significantly decrease adherence to ART regimens (Halkitis, Kutnick, Borkowski, & Parsons, 2002).

Drug-related statements elicited from participants provide further insight into dynamics of active versus non-active drug use. For example, the notion that "recovery" meant "adherence" is seen as a motivating factor for both drug abstinence and HIV medical compliance. Participants' statements revealed the use of marijuana for coping with side effects; but other statements point to the use of drugs for psychological "escape" from the reality of the HIV illness and reinforce the need for counseling and support services to this population. Participants' statements highlight the types of questions that drug users have about the interaction of drug use and HIV medications (e.g., *the impact of the drugs on the potency of the medications?; when new regimens are needed because of active drug use?*), indicating that active drug users need open discussions about the impact of drug use. Further, as reflected in the final drug-related statement, active drug users may experience conflicted thoughts about talking to physicians and other healthcare providers about their active drug use, which is similar to other findings that HIV/AIDS patients tend not to tell their providers about their non-adherence experiences (Kremer & Ironson, 2006).

Active drug use co-existing with ART is a controversial issue. Although repeated findings document drug use as compromising adherence (Uldall et al., 2004), complicating this perspective are studies that show no significant association between adherence, viral load, and current or past drug use. Stone et al. (2001) found that the complexity of medication regimens contributed to non-adherence while injection drug use did not. Among 214 participants, Martini et al. (2004) reported a high percentage of illicit drug users who complied with anti-viral therapy, suggesting "that 'drug abuse' as such is not a reliable factor for predicting compliance in patients" (p. 586). Participants in Ware et al.'s (2005) interviews revealed some regularity in occurrences of individuals taking medicines as prescribed while using drugs. Further, in response to studies finding an association between drug use and reduced viral suppression, Vlahov and Celentano (2006) suggest that the less favorable outcomes for those actively using drugs may be due *more* to their lack of adherence and service utilization than to the actual drug use per se. Nearly 40% ($n = 33$) of our participants self-reported drug and/or alcohol use while also taking HIV medications in the past 30 days; however, the extent to which drug use interferes with adherence and health outcomes is not completely clear; thus, providers should look at the range of factors as points of intervention for improving adherence as well as reducing substance abuse.

Participants' non-drug-related statements covered a broad range of reasons related to adherence, reasons that tended to fall into the same major categories as those found across other subgroups: systemic level, disease management, patient-provider relationships and individual factors. Within these categories, our findings echoed other research showing that factors such as a positive attitude, social support, and availability of services were facilitators of adherence, while issues such as side effects, complicated regiments, and fears about the medications were barriers. Further, similar to findings in other studies, housing and financial concerns were found to be of concern to our study participants. All underscore that comprehensive services are crucial to increasing successful ART outcomes. In one study, IDUs reported as much as 78% of ART use due to integration of substance abuse treatment, case management, and medical services (Mannheimer, Curtis, & El-Sadr, 1999).

Factors that emerged as needing further investigation included HCV co-infection in addition to mistrust and incarceration. Our study participants who had a co-occurring HCV infection voiced very specific concerns that uncovered fears and questions about medication interaction (e.g., *What impact are the meds having on my Hepatitis C?*). The need for providers to address these concerns is reinforced by findings that

HCV co-infection is associated with poor adherence independent of drug use (Braitstein et al., 2006). Other non-drug-related concerns point to the need to address communication and trust issues, specifically around ethno-cultural mistrust (e.g., *that nobody is paying attention to how the meds cause different side effects for different ethnic groups*). Previous studies have found ethnic/racial differences in mistrust of helping professionals and medical/social organizations as factors in engagement and retention of treatment (Longshore, Grills, Anglin, & Annon, 1997). Finally, insufficient availability of HIV meds in prisons was also raised as a concern and supports other work by Kerr et al. (2005) calling for programmatic changes to better promote optimal ART adherence in prisons.

These preliminary findings are limited by the uniqueness of our community sample and self-reported substance use. The majority of the participants were well connected to social services, including support groups. The findings contribute to the ever-existing need to unmask the realities of adherence among a group that faces substantial stigma. Research has shown that past users who are not active drug users, and even some current active users, experience adherence success (Mannheimer et al., 1999; Martini et al., 2004; Paterson et al., 2000). Thus, these findings help elucidate points of intervention to support adherence success among this group.

PRACTICE AND RESEARCH IMPLICATIONS

The statements voiced by the participants speak to two primary issues: (1) providers' need to understand the range and complexity of adherence factors beyond drug use and (2) linking participants to services that can support successful ART adherence. Obviously, substance abuse treatment is an important intervention, and certainly, transitioning from active to inactive drug use would improve general health outcomes. The fact that more than half (n = 54) of our sample did not report active drug use in the past 30 days may be reflective of the relatively large number (n = 39) who were members of a substance abuse recovery support group. Further, both drug-related and non-drug-related factors reveal potential points for intervention. Social workers and other helping professionals in health and mental health settings can help to educate and advocate for persons with dual diagnoses of HIV and substance use by working to curtail the stigma against substance users and ensure policies and practices support the rights and dignity of clients. Attending to the non-drug-related factors (social support, knowledge, and fears about the medications, strategies for dealing with side effects, mistrust, etc.) is, of course, crucial to improving adherence among this group. Providers should anticipate that clients will need assistance with coping with drug side effects and the many other day-to-day challenges facing HIV-seropositive individuals.

The participants' perceptions around adherence decision-making reveal complex aspects of their lives that should be considered in assessing a person's readiness for ART medical services. Relatively few statements (13 of 100) addressed the topic pf substance use. Instead, people living with HIV and past or current substance use appear to struggle in areas similar to those of other subgroups. Future research should further examine the relationships among the statements based on within-group differences, such as ethnicity and gender.

In sum, this paper reports on preliminary findings which were collected as part of a larger, quantitative study that will examine hierarchal relationships among the statements to further analyze sub-group patterns or clusters of perceptions about facilitators and barriers among the sample of participants. Ultimately, a better understanding of the sub-group facilitators and barriers will assist providers in their work to assess clients' readiness for ART among people living with HIV and past or current substance use. Findings from this preliminary study provided us with rich insights into the lived experience of adherence among seropositive individuals with a history of substance use. Qualitative methods allowed these individuals to use their own words in defining what facilitated or disabled adherence. In doing so, they expanded our understanding.

REFERENCES

Adam, B., Maticka-Tyndale, E., & Cohen, J. (2003). Adherence practices among people living with HIV. *AIDS Care, 15*(2), 263.

Aloisi, M. S., Arici, C., Balzano, R., Noto, P., Piscopo, R., Filice, G. et al. (2002). Behavioral correlates of adherence to antiretroviral therapy. *Journal of Acquired Immune Deficiency Syndromes, 31*, S145-S148.

Altice, F. L., Mostashari, F., & Friedland, G. H. (2001). Trust and acceptance of and adherence to antiretroviral therapy. *Journal of Acquired Immune Deficiency Syndromes, 28*, 47-58.

Arnsten, J. H., Demas, P. A., Grant, R. W., Gourevitch, M. N., Farzadegan, H., & Howard, A. A. (2002). Impact of active drug use on antiretroviral therapy adherence and viral suppression in HIV-infected drug users. JGIM: *Journal of General Internal Medicine, 17*(5), 377-381.

Bangsberg, D. R., Hecht, F. M., & Charlebois, E. D. (2000). Adherence to protease inhibitors, HIV-1 viral load, and development of drug resistance in an indigent population. *AIDS, 14,* 357-366.

Bangsberg, D. R., Hecht, F. M., Clague, H., Charlebois, E. D., Ciccarone, D., & Chesney, M. et al. (2001). Provider assessment of adherence to HIV antiretroviral therapy. *Journal of Acquired Immune Deficiency Syndromes, 26,* 435-442.

Barfod, T., Sørensen, H., Nielsen, H., Rodkjær, L., & Obel, N. (2006). 'Simply forgot' is the most frequently stated reason for missed doses of HAART irrespective of degree of adherence. *HIV Medicine, 7*(5), 285-290.

Bassetti, S., Battegay, M., & Furrer, H. (1999). Why is highly active antiretroviral therapy (HAART) not prescribed or discontinued? *Journal of Acquired Immune Deficiency Syndrome, 21,* 114-119.

Braitstein, P., Justice, A., Bangsberg, D. R., Yip, B., Alfonso, V., Schechter, M. T. et al. (2006). Hepatitis C coinfection is independently associated with decreased adherence to antiretroviral therapy in a population-based HIV cohort. *AIDS, 20* (3), 323-331.

Celentano, D., Vlahov, D., Cohn, S., Shadle, V., Obasanjo, O., & Moore, R. (1998). Self-reported antiretroviral therapy in injection drug users. *JAMA: Journal of the American Medical Association, 280*(6), 544-547.

Chesney, M. A., Ickovics, J. R., Chambers, D. B., Gifford, A. L., Neidig, J., Zwickl, B. et al. (2000b). Self-reported adherence to antiretroviral medications among participants in HIV clinical trials: The AACTG adherence instruments. *AIDS Care, 12*(3), 255-266.

Clarke, S., Delamere, S., McCullough, L., Hopkins, S., Bergin, C., & Mulcahy, F. (2003). Assessing limiting factors to the acceptance of antiretroviral therapy in a large cohort of injecting drug users. *HIV Medicine, 4*(1), 33-37.

Cook, R. L., Sereika, S. M., Hunt, S. C., Woodward, W. C., Erlen, J. A., & Conigliaro, J. (2001). Problem drinking and medication adherence among persons with HIV infection. *Journal of General Internal Medicine, 16,* 83-88.

da Silveira, V., Drachler, M., Leite, J., & Pinheiro, C. (2003). Characteristics of HIV antiretroviral regimen and treatment adherence. *The Brazilian Journal of Infectious Diseases: An Official Publication of the Brazilian Society of Infectious Diseases, 7*(3) 194-201.

Gebo, K., Keruly, J., & Moore, R. (2003). Association of social stress, illicit drug use, and health beliefs with nonadherence to antiretroviral therapy. *Journal of General Internal Medicine, 18*(2), 104-111.

Gifford, A. L., Bormann, J. E., Shively, M. J., Wright, B. C., Richman, D. D., & Bozzette, S. A. (2000). Predictors of self-reported adherence and plasma HIV concentration in patients on multidrug antiretroviral regimens. *Journal of Acquired Immune Deficiency Syndromes, 23,* 386-395.

Golin, C. E., Liu, H., Hays, R. D., Miller, L. G., Beck, C. K., Ickovics, J. et al. (2002). A prospective study of predictors of adherence to combination antiretroviral medication. *Journal of General Internal Medicine, 17,* 756-765.

Gordillo, V., Del Amo, J., & Soriano, V. (1999). Sociodemographic and psychological variables influencing adherence to antiretroviral therapy. *AIDS, 13,* 1763-1769.

Halkitis, P. N., Kutnick, A. H., Borkowski, T., & Parsons, J. T. (2002). Adherence to HIV medications and club drug use among gay and bisexual men. XIV International AIDS Conference, abstract ThPeE7856. Barcelona, Spain.

Haubrich, R. H., Little, S. J., Currier, J. S., Forthal, D. N., Kemper, C. A., Beall, G. N. et al. (1999). The value of patient-reported adherence to antiretroviral therapy in predicting virologic and immunologic response. *AIDS, 13*,1099-1107.

Ickovics, J. R., & Meade, C. S. (2002). Adherence to HAART among patients with HIV: Breakthroughs and barriers. *AIDS Care*, 14(3), 309-318.

Ingersoll, K. (2004). The impact of psychiatric symptoms, drug use, and medication regimen on non-adherence to HIV treatment. *AIDS Care, 16*(2), 199-211.

Johnson, M. O., Catz, S. L., Remien, R. H., Rotheram-Borus, M. J., Morin, S. F., Charlebois, E. et al. (2003). Theory-guided, empirically supported avenues for intervention on HIV medication nonadherence: Findings from the Healthy Living Project. *AIDS Patient Care & STDs, 17*(12), 645-656.

Johnson, M. O., Chesney, M. A., Goldstein, R. B., Remien, R. H., Catz, S., Gore-Felton, C. et al. (2006). Positive provider interactions, adherence self-efficacy, and adherence to antiretroviral medications among HIV-infected adults: A mediation model. *AIDS Patient Care & STDs, 20* (4), 258-268.

Kerr, T., Marshall, A., Walsh, J., Palepu, A. Tyndall, M., Montaner, J. et al. (2005). Determinants of HAART discontinuation among injection drug users. *AIDS Care, 17*(5), 539-549.

Kremer, H., & Ironson, G. (2006). To tell or not to tell: Why people with HIV share or don't share with their physicians whether they are taking their medications as prescribed. *AIDS Care, 18*(5), 520-528.

Longshore, D., Grills, C., Anglin, M., & Annon, K. (1997). Desire for help among African American drug users. *Journal of Drug Issues, 27*(4), 755-770.

Lucas, G. M., Cheever, L. W., Chaisson, R. E., & Moore, R. D. (2001). Detrimental effects of continued illicit drug use on the treatment of HIV-1 infection. *Journal of Acquired Immune Deficiency Syndrome, 27*, 251-259.

Malcolm, S., Ng, J., Rosen, R., & Stone, V. (2003). An examination of HIV/AIDS patients who have excellent adherence to HAART. *AIDS Care, 15*(2), 251.

Mannheimer, S., Curtis, J., & El-Sadr, W. (1999). Use of antiretroviral therapy by intravenous drug users with HIV. *JAMA: The Journal of The American Medical Association, 281*(8) 700.

Martini M., Recchia E., Nasta P., Castanotto D., Chiaffarino F., Parazzini F. et al. (2004). Illicit drug use: Can it predict adherence to antiretroviral therapy? *European Journal of Epidemiology, 19*(6 (Print)), 585-587.

Mellins, C. A., Kang, E., Leu, C., Havens, J., & Chesney, M. (2003). Longitudinal study of mental health and psychosocial predictors of medical treatment adherence in mothers living with HIV disease. *AIDS Patient Care and STDs, 17*, 407-416.

Montessori, V., Press, N., Harris, M., Akagi, L., & Montaner, J. (2004). Adverse effects of antiretroviral therapy for HIV infection. *CMAJ: Canadian Medical Association Journal = Journal De L'association Medicale Canadienne, 170*(2 [Print]), 229-238.

Oggins, J. (2003). Notions of HIV and Medication among Multiethnic People Living with HIV. *Health & Social Work, 28*(1), 53.

Paterson, D. L., Swindells, S., Mohr, J., Brester, M., Vergis, E. M., Squier, C. et al. (2000). Adherence to protease inhibitor therapy and outcomes in patients with HIV infection. *Annals Internal Medicine, 133*, 21-30.

Power, R., Koopman, C., Volk, J., Israelski, D.M., Stone, L., Chesney, M. A. et al. (2003). Social support, substance use, and denial in relationship to antiretroviral treatment adherence among HIV-infected persons. *AIDS Patient Care & STDs, 17*(5), 245-252.

Prentiss, D. E., Balmas, M. G., Power, R., & Israelski, D. M. (2002). Use of marijuana among people with HIV and its relationship to adherence to antiretroviral treatment, use of alternative therapies and complete viral suppression in a public health care setting in northern California. *XIV International AIDS Conference*, abstract WePeB6008. Barcelona, Spain.

Read, T., Mijch, A., & Fairley, C. (2003). Adherence to antiretroviral therapy: Are we doing enough? *Internal Medicine Journal*, 33(5/6), 254-256.

Reback, C. J., Larkins, S., & Shoptaw, S. (2003). *AIDS Care, 15*(6), 775-785.

Sorensen, J., Mascovich, A., Wall, T., Dephilippis, D., Batki, S., & Chesney, M. (1998). Medication adherence strategies for drug abusers with HIV/AIDS. *AIDS Care, 10*(3), 297-312.

Stone, V. E., Hogan, J. W., & Schuman, P. (2001). Antiretroviral regimen complexity, self-reported adherence, and HIV patients' understanding of their regimens: survey of women in the HER study. *Journal of Acquired Immune Deficiency Syndrome, 28*, 124-131.

Trochim, W. (1989). An introduction to concept mapping for planning and evaluation. *Evaluation and Program Planning, 12*(1), 1-16.

Tucker, J., Burnam, M., Sherbourne, C., Kung, F., & Gifford, A. (2003). Substance use and mental health correlates of nonadherence to antiretroviral medications in a sample of patients with human immunodeficiency virus infection. *American Journal of Medicine, 114*(7), 573.

Turner, B., Fleishman, J. A., Wenger, N., London, A. S., Burnam, M. A., & Shapiro, M. F., (2001). Effects of drugs abuse and mental disorders on use and type of antiretroviral therapy in HIV-infected persons. *Journal of General Internal Medicine, 16*, 625-633.

Uldall, K., Palmer, N., Whetten, K., & Mellins, C. (2004). Adherence in people living with HIV/AIDS, mental illness, and chemical dependency: A review of the literature. *AIDS Care, 16*, S71-S96.

Vlahov, D., & Celentano, D. (2006). Access to highly active antiretroviral therapy for injection drug users: Adherence, resistance, and death. *Cadernos De Saúde Pública/ Ministério Da Saúde, Fundaçno Oswaldo Cruz, Escola Nacional De Saúde Pública*, 22(4 [Print]), 705-718.

Wagner, J. H., Justice, A. C., Chesney, M., Sinclair, G., Weissman, S., & Rodriguez-Barradas, M. (2001). Patient and provider-reported adherence: toward a clinically useful approach to measuring antiretroviral adherence. *Journal of Clinical Epidemiology, 54*, S91-S98.

Ware, N., Wyatt, M., & Tugenberg, T. (2005). Adherence, stereotyping and unequal HIV treatment for active users of illegal drugs. *Social Science & Medicine, 61*(3), 565-576.

doi:10.1300/J187v06n01_10

Index